Having A Baby:
An Experience Of A Lifetime

Having A Baby:
An Experience Of A Lifetime

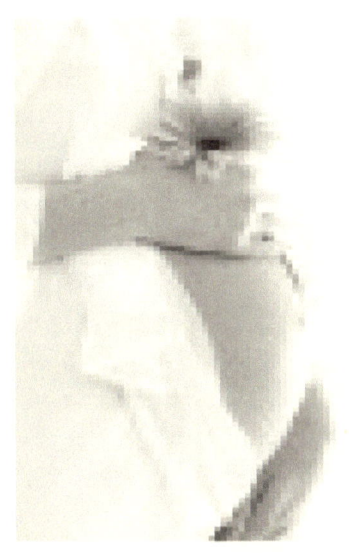

BY

Emmanuel C. Mba

To order additional copies of this book, contact:
Xlibris Corporation
1-888-795-4274
www.Xlibris.com
Orders@Xlibris.com
81017

CONTENTS

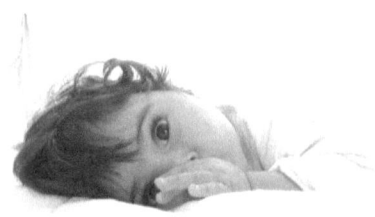

INTRODUCTION

Life, as you know it, is about to change. Perhaps you have dreamed about this pregnancy since you were a child, toddling about with dolls in a nurturing fashion. Or maybe you had to lift your jaw up off the floor after your home pregnancy test came back with a highly unexpected positive result. Either way, this huge event begins a whole new chapter in your life. Having a baby changes everything about what you are: physically, socially, morally, *everything*. You will continually be amazed at your strength, your uncanny ability to work through extreme exhaustion, and by the awesome and sometimes otherworldly love you feel for your baby.

Get ready to be given advice by everyone who is aware of your pregnancy, and once you start showing don't be surprised if complete strangers brazenly insist upon not only offering unsolicited advice but also regaling you with horrific stories of painful childbirth. It's just what experienced (and not so experienced) moms do to other moms . . . consider it your proper hazing and accept it with a grain of salt.

Unless you stumbled upon the discovery of your expectant status late in the game, you can take solace in the fact that you have some time to prepare. Although it is true that no amount of advice can truly prepare you for everything that is about to happen there is something to be said for taking in as much information as you can. Knowledge is power, after all, and knowing all you can will certainly make you feel a little better about what you're about to leap into.

A word of caution about the aforementioned importance of learning all you can about having a baby. Information is great, but too much information can leave an expectant parent's mind swimming in a vast sea of "what if?" which will surely cause much more harm than good. Realize that your body is going to feel as though it is rebelling against you most of the time, and every single twitch or ache is certainly not indicative of a crisis. It is good to know the sorts of signs which merit your attention, but don't spend countless nights combing through chapters in baby books which detail everything that can go wrong. Remember that the vast majority of pregnancies result in normal deliveries and healthy babies. Do not add extra stress to your already stressed mind and body by spending your time worrying about what might happen. Take a deep breath, enjoy your pregnancy, and get ready for the impending whirlwind.

THE CALM BEFORE THE STORM

If you are reading this before even getting pregnant then congratulations to you on being the kind of proactive person who plans everything ahead of time. Now for the brutal truth: pregnancy and childbirth are things, which you can plan for until the cows come home but things hardly ever go as planned. You may intend on working a full-time job right up to the week before having the baby only to find out in week twenty of your pregnancy that you need to go on strict bed rest. Or maybe you have everything planned out just perfectly for your new addition and then you're told you're carrying twins. Don't be dismayed; pregnancy and childbirth are probably among the most amazing feats you will ever accomplish. Just try to roll with the punches. Having said that, there are some things you can do to ready yourself for your impending pregnancy attempts.

PHYSICAL READINESS

Ask your doctor for a preconception checkup. If you let your doctor in on the secret that you'll be trying to get pregnant soon then he or she can do a full work-up of blood work and other tests to make sure your body is ready for the physical strain of pregnancy. Some doctors prescribe prenatal vitamins to women who are planning on getting pregnant.

Now is the time to start eating well and getting rest. You may as well get into the habit beforehand of taking in nutritious foods and avoiding junk while also making sure you get the sort of rest you need. This will make it easier to eat right and rest well during pregnancy.

Genetic counseling is available, but expensive.
Some people have very valid reasons for seeking out genetic counseling because there are certain diseases and ailments whose odds of showing up in your baby can increase exponentially if both partners carry the traits in their genes.

If you have anything like sickle cell anemia or cystic fibrosis in your family then it may be worth it to seek out genetic counseling with your spouse. The counselor will check out both of you and let you know the likelihood of you conceiving a child who will be born with something like this.

EMOTIONAL READINESS

Having a baby does not solve marital issues. If anything, having a baby will usually put a huge strain on the relationship. So if the main goal is to get closer to your spouse or to try to save a failing marriage then maybe counseling is the answer, but bringing a baby into an already volatile situation is not the solution by any means.

Are you ready for a huge change in your life? You need to realize that life does not simply chug along as usual after you have a baby. You will be making huge changes and noticeable sacrifices when the baby is born. Are you ready to make this sort of commitment?

SIGNS THAT YOU'RE PREGNANT

If you have spent a great deal of time trying to get pregnant than you know that oftentimes the beginnings of the menstrual cycle can seem deceivingly like a new pregnancy. Pregnancy books tell hopeful mothers to be on the lookout for tender breasts, fatigue, and moodiness, but as women know all these signs can also simply point to just another appearance from The Monthly Visitor. Some women who are trying to conceive follow a similar disappointing pattern every month where they will swear that they "feel" pregnant, only to start another period and another missed opportunity to successfully conceive. This same pattern, month after month, can wear down even the most tenacious woman.

Luckily, not all women go through this emotional rollercoaster. Some women get pregnant the very first month they try, while others wind up pregnant without every really having tried. There is no way to tell for absolute certain if you are pregnant without a blood test from your doctor, but there are some tell-tale signs which can tip you off that there may be a bun in the oven.

PHYSICAL SIGNS

Be aware that every single so-called sign of pregnancy can be caused by something else entirely, and it is always best to consult a doctor to confirm a pregnancy. A combination of these signs along with an active attempt at getting pregnant, though, makes for pretty good odds.

There's no period. If you have been tracking your period every month and you are usually pretty regular the absence of your period is a pretty good indicator that something is going on. Women who are not attempting to get pregnant and who are currently on birth control are certainly not immune to pregnancy as no birth control except for abstinence is fail-safe. Any missed period merits the purchase of a home pregnancy test, just to be sure.

You have to pee like a racehorse. During pregnancy there are so many wacky hormones shooting through a woman's body that a lot of things change. A pregnant woman's bladder needs to empty more often, particularly in the first and third trimester. Make sure you always know where a clean restroom is when you're out in public.

You really need a nap. Creating a whole new being isn't easy work for a body so there is no surprise to the fact that pregnancy can bring with it sheer exhaustion, even early on. Try to indulge the urge to sleep whenever you can because once the baby comes you won't be getting nearly as much sleep as you can now.

Everything smells icky. If you walk into the grocery store and everything suddenly repulses you, it may be time to pick up a home pregnancy test along with your groceries. Although this feeling will eventually pass, many women say that the icky-smell problem is the one that tipped them off to being pregnant.

You're starving. Some women never feel nauseous in early pregnancy, but instead want to eat everything in sight. It takes extra calories to build a baby, so this makes sense. Don't be shocked if you feel nauseous early on and then ravenous later in the pregnancy.

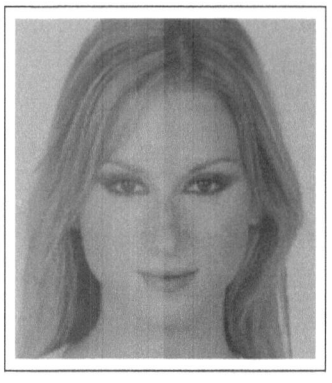

You're freezing / you're on fire.
Body temperature is regulated differently in a pregnant woman's body. Grabbing a jacket or fanning yourself while everyone else is comfortable can be an indicator that something is different in your body. Dressing in layers can help you if this becomes a constant issue through your pregnancy because you can add or subtract clothing as needs be.

Your breasts are bigger. They are probably a little sore too. This is only one change in a series of many which your breasts will go through during the pregnancy and throughout breastfeeding, should you choose to do it.

EMOTIONAL SIGNS

As with physical changes, every emotional change associated with pregnancy can easily be attributed to something else, such as stress or depression. There are some women who start to realize they are pregnant after their significant other asks them if they have gone completely insane.

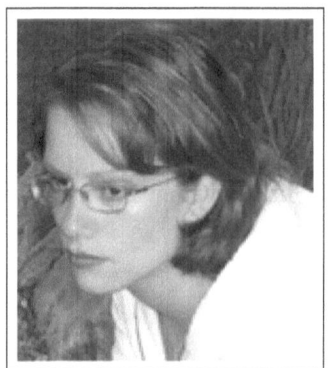

You're crying like there's no tomorrow. Chalk this up to hormones accompanied by the fatigue you may be experiencing. If what you thought was PMS doesn't go away and that period never starts, you're probably pregnant.

You're cranky. Even though you may not yet realize it, your body is working furiously to create a new baby. As with the aforementioned crying, crankiness and moodiness may be a result of the fatigue and the hormonal changes your body is going through.

Something just feels different. There are some women who claim to simply "feel" pregnant. It's true that there are some women who are so in tune with their bodies that they can just sense that there is a pregnancy going on even before a home pregnancy test can identify a positive result.

There are dozens of other signs that can point to a pregnancy. Some unfortunate women seem to inherit every single pregnancy malady possible and of course realize they are pregnant when everything aches and they are puking up every single meal. Other women have such subtle signs that they really need to pay attention to their bodies to get the message. Most women, however, have a combination of pregnancy signals and eventually realize that all signs are pointing to a pregnancy.

YOUR EVER CHANGING BODY

No matter what stage of pregnancy you are currently in, you need to realize that your body simply doesn't belong to you any more, or at least for the time being. Women look at the changes in their bodies with wonderment, amusement, or horror. Luckily, not every woman gets every single possibly change that may come with pregnancy. That would be one miserable woman indeed. Every woman is blessedly different, though, and your body's reaction to the pregnancy depends on several different factors including genetic predisposition, current health status, and environmental factors.

THE GOOD

You're glowing!
Pregnancy hormones coupled with the vast nutrients contained in prenatal vitamins can result in shinier and thicker hair, stronger fingernails, and for some women a nice complexion. There

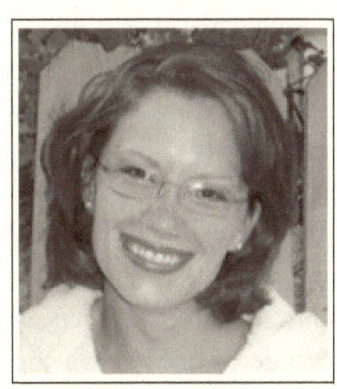

are some women who take to pregnancy so beautifully that they have a certain glow about them, almost like an aura of motherly content. Now of course there are countless jokes that could be inserted here about how that motherly glow will likely vanish with the first real painful contraction, but for now it's best for women to just enjoy their pregnant radiance.

It's Obvious. When your belly bump comes in and it is obvious that you are pregnant you will be surprised how many people come to your aid. Strangers will open doors for you, passengers give up their seats on the bus, and everyone is just more willing to be helpful. This is to your physical advantage because everyone sees your condition; you may not be the kind of person who is willing to slow down and listen to your body, but with everyone around you cautioning you to take it easy you may have to actually listen.

Yay! No period to contend with! Unless you have one of the rare pregnancies which involve periodic bleeding then you will be quite happy to get rid of your monthly flow for the entire duration of your pregnancy. There is nothing quite like a vacation from your period and it almost makes the discomforts of pregnancy worth it. When will your period return? Immediately after having your baby you'll have a post-delivery period, which can involve some really dramatic bleeding which can make even the heartiest woman a little queasy. This is simply your body cleaning out all the stuff it no longer needs. After this stint of bleeding concludes you may find a normal period resumes pretty quickly, but if you're breastfeeding your baby it can take much longer for your period to start back up. Some lucky women go beyond a year post-delivery without a period, thanks to nursing their baby.

THE BAD

Are you feeling like a stuffed sausage? For some women, the act of swelling and bloating is simply par for the course with pregnancy. After all, it isn't only your stomach, which is going to get bigger. Pregnancy fundamentally changes your body whether you like it or not, and it isn't uncommon for women to actually go up a shoe size from bloating and swelling during pregnancy. Don't be shocked if a year or so after pregnancy you look at a picture of your pregnant self and don't even recognize the swollen face in the photo. Drinking plenty of water, ironically, can help keep swelling at bay because it helps flush everything out of your system. Be advised, though, that rapid swelling is something that needs to be checked by your doctor because it can be a sign of problems. If your doctor finds no problems and you continue to swell just rest assured that even if your ankles disappear while your pregnant they will more than likely magically reappear quickly after you give birth. It's amazing how quickly the body can recover after the baby is born.

You can't poop. Your internal workings slow down when you're pregnant, and this includes your digestive system. Add to this the fact that prenatal vitamins have a ton of iron in them to stave off anemia issues, and you're bound to be . . . well . . . bound. Sometimes a pregnancy can bring with it a double whammy of constipation and hemorrhoids, which really makes bowel movements uncomfortable. So not only do you have problems mustering up the need to poop, but the act of pooping can be incredibly painful. Luckily doctors can prescribe stool softeners, and hemorrhoid wipes, which are sold in stores, do a good job of cooling the pain after a bowel movement. On a depressing note, once you get hemorrhoids they may shrink down but they never go away even after the baby is born unless you have hemorrhoid removal surgery. Hemorrhoid removal surgery is no walk in the park, and although patients say it helps tremendously after they heal they also say that the first bowel movement after the surgery sort of feels like pooping shattered glass. Ouch.

Do you feel like you're burping up food all the time? Acid reflux is common with women in late pregnancy since the baby is pressing up on the digestive system, making it difficult for everything to run smoothly. How do you know if you have acid reflux? If you have burps that feel sort of like a small bit of stomach acid has invaded your throat, then it's likely you're having this problem. Sometimes it can be so bad that pregnant women will abruptly awaken from a deep sleep, coughing and gasping for air accompanied by the disgusting feeling of having thrown up a little in their throat. There are some medications, which are safe to use for acid reflux during pregnancy, but many times it can be easily controlled with dietary changes. You will quickly realize which foods result in grief, and you can either avoid them all together or simply eat them early in the day long before laying down to go to sleep. Some common culprits include tomato sauce, coffee, and citrus fruits. If acid reflux becomes a real problem then talk to your doctor; there is no reason to suffer if you don't have to. Acid reflux is another ailment that seems to magically disappear once the baby is born, so just know that you won't be burping up spaghetti sauce for the rest of your life.

Do you feel a bit wobbly? Even before you belly starts to expand you may find that your balance feels a little off. This is truly the time to put away your heels and trade them in for some sensible shoes because your balance is going to disappoint you time and again during pregnancy. When you begin to show, and when you can no longer see your feet, you are really going to need to pay attention to what you're doing and take care to not fall down stairs or trip on rugged terrain. Remind yourself daily that you are in a delicate state, and act accordingly.

THE UGLY

Is that a roadmap on your belly? Not all women get stretch marks on their pregnant bellies, but there are a good amount of women who do. Really, there is only so much your poor skin can take before it starts forming stretch marks, and the average pregnant belly gets pretty darn big. You'll notice stretch marks at first, as red marks, which look a lot, like scratches. They'll get longer and more defined the bigger your belly gets. Even after the baby is born and the belly begins to return back to its normal size your stretch marks will remain. They'll start to fade eventually, and instead of being a blazing red color they will instead look a more silvery color. So they'll never really go away naturally, but they won't be nearly as pronounced as they once were. Are there ways to avoid getting stretch marks in pregnancy? There are many creams and lotions on the market which purport to prevent stretch marks but nothing has ever been proven. If you wind up with stretch marks try to see them as an earned badge and consider purchasing a one-piece bathing suit next summer instead of a bikini.

Are those craters on your face? If you thought acne breakouts were reserved for puberty and certain times of the month then you'll be disappointed to find out that many pregnant women break out with acne pretty regularly. Chalk this on up to hormones. If the acne bothers you then be sure to check with your doctor before employing an acne remedy. Some acne medicine is simply not appropriate for a pregnant woman to use.

What are those veins on my legs? While you're pregnant you can see your veins through your skin easier, so this can result in all sorts of interesting bluish patterns emerging just below your skin. Some pregnant women also have problems with varicose veins that are not only unsightly but also painful in some instances. Staying off your feet and not gaining too much weight can help you avoid varicose veins, and as far as being able to see your veins easier that will go away shortly after having the baby, if not before then.

Sure, pregnancy can feel downright miserable at times. There are other times, though, when you will find yourself patting your belly and smiling to yourself about how amazing you feel. If you begin to feel overwhelmed with the changes to your body then remind yourself that you are busy growing life, and if this means you need to be uncomfortable for a while then so be it. Many of the discomforts of pregnancy magically dissolve the moment you have the baby . . . it's one of the gifts of childbirth. Just remember to cut yourself some slack; too often in our society pregnant women are expected to virtually ignore their condition and continue on with their daily tasks without getting the rest they need and deserve. Rest up now, because after the baby comes it's a whole new ballgame.

EATING FOR TWO

Most pregnant women get awfully hungry at some point of their pregnancy. It's no wonder since their bodies are working overtime to produce a perfect little bundle of joy. Problems arise, however, when women use pregnancy as justification for stuffing their face with everything their heart desires. They suppose that if their bodies are screaming for a twelve layer chocolate cake then they must certainly have a deficiency of something that is in chocolate cake . . . magnesium perhaps? The truth of the matter is that during pregnancy a woman's body only needs to take in an additional 300 calories on average, and that's probably the equivalent of a couple of bites of a decadent cake. Yes, listen to your body, but don't go crazy. Remember the important fact that you're going to have to one-day work to lose this weight; it doesn't all just magically melt off when the baby is born.

FOOD CRAVINGS

Pregnancy cravings go beyond pickles and ice cream. Although no one is entirely sure what causes a pregnant woman to have intense food cravings, the general consensus is that mineral and vitamin deficiencies play a role. In this sense the body is alerting the pregnant woman of a lack of something and is begging for an appropriate food product to restore the balance. This theory makes sense for the most part, but many pregnant women find themselves craving items with little or no nutritional value, so this blows the theory right out of the water. Is it merely a caloric necessity? Or perhaps raging hormones play a part? For whatever reason, do not be surprised if one day you are suddenly and indescribably held captive by an immediate need for a really ridiculous food.

Gimme that sandwich! One woman shared a story where she demanded her husband make a three-hour drive to get a pork barbeque sandwich from a little café. She would accept no substitute and also would not take no for an answer. Finally, exhausted by the nagging, the husband made the trip and returned six hours later, bearing the prized pork sandwich. When she saw that he had neglected to purchase the café's prized sauce in addition to the sandwich she burst into tears and refused to eat it. She never did get to satisfy her craving because at this point the husband was near tears himself and wasn't going to attempt another trip. Today they laugh about it, but at the time it felt like the end of the world to her.

FOOD AVERSIONS

Sometimes everything just seems gross. There may come a time in your pregnancy when you just can't stand the sight and smell of food. This occurs particularly in the first trimester when hormones are really hopping. There have been a few theories proposed to explain why pregnant women sometimes have food aversions, but perhaps the most plausible theory involves a pregnant woman's heightened sense of smell. Repulsion to certain foods is supposed to be the pregnant body's way of guarding against spoiled foods and sometimes this defense just seems to go haywire. So even if a food is perfectly fit for consumption it may still make you fell ill.

Some food aversions aren't joking around. There are some pregnant women who simply can't cook, grocery shop, or even talk about food without eventually running to the bathroom to throw up. Luckily this doesn't last through the whole pregnancy for most women, so if you find yourself overwhelmed by smells when entering a restaurant or disgusted by food presented before you just know that this probably won't last the whole time. If, however, you find that you simply can't keep any food down and you aren't gaining any weight then it is time to have a talk with your doctor.

EATING RIGHT

Have a plan. Some women have one certain item they use as their "Craving Buster" so if they find themselves desperate for a huge box of cookies they will instead turn to their usual glass of milk or fruit smoothie. The trick is to get something on your stomach so that the caloric need is fulfilled without giving in to a huge sweet tooth attack. Sure, it feels like this is the only time in your life when you can pig out and people won't think anything except, "look at that cute pregnant lady with the big belly over there." Just remember that big bellies aren't quite so cute anymore after the baby has been born.

Moderation is the key. Do you want a cookie? Okay, have a cookie, but don't eat twelve of them. Many women go through their pregnancies indulging in something every day and that's just fine as long as it is in moderation. Yes, pregnancy can be miserable, and yes, sometimes the only thing that can bring a smile to your face is a big candy bar. Everyone understands the need for a pregnant woman to indulge herself once in a while. You'll have less risk of problems, however, if you attempt to stay healthy before labor. So this means that you pay attention to your body and get your extra calories without laying waste to a donut shop.

Everything you eat winds up in your baby's belly. That means if you down twelve coffees a day then your little baby is learning very early on what caffeine is like. Some researchers suggest that the foods a pregnant woman eats can have a direct effect on what sorts of foods a baby likes after being born. Now is the time to load up on vegetables and fruits in an attempt to not only supply your baby with nutritious foods, but also to get them used to the flavors.

If you leaped into pregnancy with the expectation of being able to gorge yourself to your heart's content you'll be saddened to realize that this practice is generally frowned upon by doctors. Yes, there is room for some indulgence when it comes to eating during pregnancy, but you must realize that gaining weight from food while pregnant is just like gaining weight while not pregnant. In other words, when you go through labor the weight you lose is going to be the weight of the baby and the surrounding amniotic fluid, not the weight you gained from eating pie every night. That weight will have to be lost the old fashioned way. Take care to not go overboard.

PLANNING FOR THE BIG DAY

The day is rapidly approaching when you can finally meet the baby you have carried in your body and dreamed about for so long. You probably have a strong desire to hold your baby, gaze lovingly into your baby's eyes, and to sing sweet lullabies to your precious angel. All beautiful fantasies aside, though, it's important to research and plan how you would like the big day to go. If you show up to deliver your baby without any sort of plan in place you're at the mercy of the whims of the hospital staff, and sometimes that's not a good place to be.

GET READY . . .

Your partner can be your rock. There are going to be some times when you're pregnant where you feel awfully overwhelmed. These are the times when you should turn to your spouse for some support, both emotional and physical. Hopefully you have the sort of spouse who helps you without being asked, who insists that you rest and relax, and who doesn't mind dealing with your inevitable exhaustion and mood swings. If your spouse is less than intuitive with your needs then now is the time to realize that he probably isn't a mind reader and you need to let your desires known. Don't sit and simmer angrily that he isn't doing the dishes without you asking him; ask him to do the dishes and he'll probably do them.

Some women go it alone. Some women jump into single motherhood by choice, while others are forced to go through pregnancy and parenting alone due to unavoidable circumstances. If you are this type of woman, then hopefully you have a solid support system through your family, friends, or even through a church community. Having children is no simple task, even when you have a dedicated partner helping you. Rest assured that there are countless women who do have children on their own and who do a darn good job of it, it's just twice as hard as it would be otherwise. A woman facing the trials and tribulations of parenthood without a partner should not be reluctant to take people up on offers for help, and certainly shouldn't be afraid to ask for help either. You may not be Superwoman, but you're pretty close if you can pull off motherhood effectively without a partner.

A birthing plan is a good idea. The birthing plan is the plan, which lets everyone in on what the mother-to-be wants on the big day. That includes any sort of environmental factors such as music playing or particular decorations in the room, and should also include specific instructions to the caring of your newborn. Do you want to breastfeed exclusively? Make sure the birthing plan includes no bottles of formula for the baby. Do you want to hold your baby before they weigh and clean him? If your doctor allows this practice, then it should be specified in the birthing plan.

Where do you want to have the baby? The locations available for having your baby go way beyond the labor and delivery wing of your local hospital. Some women are uncomfortable with sterile and medicinal setting of a hospital and instead opt for a birthing center. Birthing centers are generally staffed by midwives and do not offer certain things like epidurals or emergency care. If you have a normal, low-risk pregnancy and the idea of having your baby in a more natural setting suits you then look into a birthing center. Since emergencies can arise, however, it is best to pick a birthing center which is located near a hospital. You can even choose to go through labor in the comfort of your own home, as many women do. Some women have their babies at home with the assistance of a midwife, sometimes even giving birth while in their own bathtubs. This may sound appealing to you, but it is important to remember that labor hurts . . . a lot. Your first baby may not be the time to plan a home birth with candles lit and faerie music playing in the background. Perhaps it is best to save that for subsequent births when you have a better idea of what you're getting yourself into and have a better understanding of your pain threshold.

You'll get to know your doctor pretty well. During your pregnancy you will probably see your doctor once a month, even if you're feeling well. These doctor visits allow for the doctor to monitor your progress and give you a chance to barrage the doctor with all the questions which have been swirling around in your head since the last visit. Don't be shy about asking any questions which may arise . . . doctors have heard it all and you probably can't think of a single question which hasn't already been discussed in that office. As your pregnancy progresses you will be scheduled for appointments twice a month, until you finally end up with weekly appointments in your final month. Be sure you have a doctor who you like a trust because you're going to be seeing an awful lot of him or her in the coming months.

Enjoy the parties and the gift registries. Many expectant parents choose to register for the gifts they need instead of simply just letting their friends and family arbitrarily decide for them. This is a great idea since people who have never had children probably don't have the faintest idea of what new parents need, but the funny thing is that often times it's true that expectant parents have no idea of what they need either. When you're shopping for items on your registry try to let practicality lead you instead of oohing and aahing over cutesy outfits and adorable decorative items. Look instead to diapers and wipes, blankets and spit-ups rags, and things like baby monitors or baby carriers. Keep in mind that certain items which usually show up on baby registries such as high chairs, safety gates, and even teething rings are all things which will not be needed for at least a couple of months. It's a much better idea to register for the items you will need right after the baby is born. Do be sure, however, to throw in some cute toys or outfits to appease the people shopping with your registry because although practical items are great many people honestly just get a real kick out of buying cute baby stuff.

Ultrasounds can be a lot of fun. Even if you aren't able to get one of the new high-definition ultrasounds done you will still have a lot of fun sneaking a glance at your baby before he is born. How much you will be able to see depends greatly on when the ultrasound is done. Some doctors do ultrasounds right off the bat if they are having trouble hearing a heartbeat or if there is some other reason. Most pregnant women get ultrasounds done closer to twenty-five weeks or later because this allows the technician to check all the vital organs, the growth of the baby, and in some cases they can tell you if you're having a boy or girl. Some expectant mothers find out for the first time during an ultrasound that they are expecting more than one baby! Babies can be spied sucking their thumbs, waving their arms, or even doing movements, which look an awful lot like dancing during the ultrasounds. Seeing your baby is a great confirmation of what is going on inside your swelling baby. Usually you will leave the appointment with a nice little blurry picture of your baby, which you will cherish long after the baby, is born. Some stores even sell frames, which are made specifically for ultrasound pictures. A word of caution regarding those companies, which offer high-resolution ultrasounds independent of a doctor: these companies aren't medically staffed and therefore are doing these ultrasounds only because there is a market for them. You should be leery of utilizing their services, especially if having an ultrasound through them makes you less vigilant about having an ultrasound with a qualified technician.

Do you want to know the gender of your baby? Some researchers suggest that women who do not find out the sex of their baby actually tend to push harder during labor because they are just that anxious to see what gender the baby is. Many expectant parents like the element of surprise attached to not knowing what the baby will be, and still other superstitious parents feel that the only thing they should worry about is if the baby is healthy or not.

On the other hand there is certainly something to be said for knowing if you're having a boy or a girl so you can plan accordingly. Green and yellow neutral outfits and decorations are cute, but some parents long to buy the definitive blue or pink. If you and your spouse are at an impasse about whether to find out the baby's gender or not then maybe you should come to a compromise such as the mom deciding with the first baby and the dad to decide with the next baby. Some would argue the ultimate decision rests with the mom since she's the one carrying the baby, but of course some men would disagree.

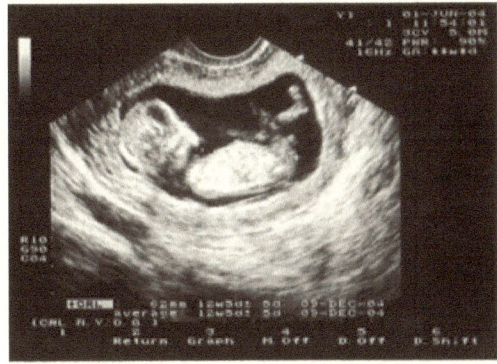

SET . . .

Do you want a big crowd or an intimate affair? Some women allow massive amounts of people into the room, cameras in hand, ready to witness the birth. Other women opt for the spouse and the medical staff, and that's it. It all depends on the wishes of the pregnant woman and the rules and regulations of the hospital or birthing center. Be sure to ask the doctor before planning a veritable family reunion in your room. You can also take comfort in knowing that if your pushy mother-in-law shows up while you're in labor it's pretty easy to whisper to the nurse to get her out of the room. Labor and delivery staff are used to these sorts of situations and aren't afraid to kick someone out of the room. As a bonus you can later blame it on the nurse so you don't have to take blame for your mother-in-law missing the actual birthing process. One nurse was famous for yelling out, "If you weren't there for the conception, then you won't be there for the birth!" to clear the delivery room of relatives.

What in the world is a doula? A doula is essentially a birthing coach. She is someone who is trained on making the birthing mother comfortable during labor and can also act as the mom's advocate. You hire a doula well before going into labor and discuss with her in detail what you are looking for with your birthing experience, and it is her job to make it happen. While you're in labor your doula will make sure everything goes according to your birthing plan and will also use different methods in an attempt to make your labor go smoothly. Some doulas will utilize massage techniques while others will help with breathing exercises. Basically, you are paying her to do everything a female village elder might have done in the past. She is there to hold your hand and keep you calm. Some husbands are threatened by a doula since husbands want so desperately to comfort their wives when they are in pain, while other husbands welcome any sort of help. If the idea of a doula appeals to you then make sure you check her references extensively before signing a contract with her . . . the last thing you need is to be in labor and then have your doula either cheerfully announce this is the first birth she has ever attended or worse yet to have her pass out from the sight of blood.

Now is the time to have a little fun. You may feel tired from the pregnancy and perhaps the last thing on your mind is a date night with your spouse. The unfortunate truth is that the exhaustion you're experiencing right now most likely does not even compare to the mind-numbing exhaustion some new parents experience after the baby is born. For this reason you may want to consider going out on the town a little more than you're used to because after the baby is born doing things like running out to see a movie or for a bite to eat will become distant memories, at least for a while. Don't use the pregnancy as an excuse to sit at home and sulk about all the things you can't do because before you know it you'll have a newborn baby and you'll be wondering to yourself why you didn't take advantage of the time you had before the baby was born. Just be sure that while you're living it up and having fun you're not indulging in alcohol or tobacco products for obvious reasons.

Naming a child is a big responsibility. You should grant absolute power to your spouse to veto any name he doesn't like, just as you should have the same power with names he likes. It doesn't matter if you have been on love with a certain name since you were a little girl. If your spouse thinks the name is horrible then just drop it. Try buying a big book of baby names and then go through it highlighting the names you like and then have your partner go through and highlight the names he likes. After you have finished with the highlighting go back and check out any of the names which you both highlighted, and then go from there. Also be sure to take into consideration other factors before deciding on a name. Are the men in your family slight of build? Don't name your son Zeus. Do the females in your family have a propensity towards being big-boned with facial hair? Don't name your daughter Juliet. Also, take care to not name your baby the same name which everyone else is naming their kids. There are plenty of resources which will tell you what the most popular names of the past few years have been. Try to avoid anything in the top ten because even though kids don't like to be named something bizarre they also don't want to be one of four kids with the same name in school.

Do you want to name your baby before he is born? Some parents go so far as to name their babies before they are born, adorning the nursery with personalized blankets and trinkets. Unless there is a custom in your family of naming a child an ancestral name then it is a good idea to wait to announce the name of your baby until after he is born. Not only does this avoid possible conflicts, such as a relative naming their baby the same name before yours is born thus resulting in a huge family feud, but sometimes a baby just doesn't suit the name they are intended to have. It is best to have a short list of possible names when going to the hospital and decide on the baby's name after you lay eyes on him. More often than not your baby will match your favorite name just fine.

Do you have pets? If you have dogs with aggressive tendencies it may be time now to find new homes for them. No matter how much you adore these dogs you will undoubtedly adore your baby more, and it simply isn't worth the risk. If your dog isn't normally aggressive then you need to make the decision whether the dog will be able to handle the new addition and act accordingly. Even cats can create a problem when a new baby arrives by trying to cuddle up with the baby in the crib or even by attacking the baby.

If you can't train your cat to stay out of the crib and to not lash out at your baby then your cat needs a new home, pure and simple. No matter how passionate you are about your pets, even if they have always been treated like your children in the past you need to take into account the fact that animals are unpredictable around babies, and especially when big changes occur in the home. Don't make the mistake of creating a volatile situation.

GO!

Most women recognize contractions. Contractions range from a tightening feeling to a full-on painful ache, which starts small, gets huge, and then eventually winds down. So many women worry that they won't realize they are having contractions but the truth is that this is unlikely. Most women who are going through their first labor experience will have contractions for quite some time before they are ever dilated enough to start pushing, so don't panic if you have a contraction which feels pretty intense. In reality, they're probably going to get worse . . . much worse, as a matter of fact. You should discuss with your doctor at what point he or she would like for you to head to the hospital; typically the doctor will say that— when the contractions get hard enough to where you can't talk through them and they also come in regular intervals then it's time to head in to get checked out. One more thing you should know about contractions: although it is disappointing for the eager mom-to-be, you may head into the maternity ward and get checked only to find out you are hardly dilated. If you're sent home to labor some more, try not to get discouraged. Now would be a good time to start rolling the video camera so you can get video of you bracing yourself through contractions. It makes for excellent guilt material when your child is older.

Whoosh! Not all women experience their water breaking before they go into labor. In fact, many first-time moms wind up having their water broken by their doctor using a hook device, which ruptures the amniotic sack. The process isn't as uncomfortable as it sounds; so don't worry if your doctor has to do it. For the other women who actually experience water breaking naturally, the actual event can vary. Some women wake up and initially think that they have accidentally peed in their sleep. Others are in the middle of some daily task when all of a sudden they look down and there is a big wet spot. In some instances, a woman may not have felt a single contraction and then all of a sudden their water breaks and the contractions start coming quickly. Whatever the situation, water breaking is always a good reason to call the doctor. More than likely the doctor will say to head to the hospital since the risk of infection is greater once the water has broken. That means that you shouldn't mess around and lollygag . . . just put on a sanitary napkin to catch the fluid and grab your suitcase.

Are there any women who don't realize they're in labor? There are token stories of women who don't feel strong contractions and don't realize they are in labor until all of a sudden they get the urge to push. These stories complement nicely the urban myths of women not knowing they are pregnant until they suddenly go into labor. Although there have certainly been actual accounts of these sorts of instances they are extremely rare and aren't really something you should be too concerned with. Of for one reason or another you get the distinct feeling that you are in labor but there are no physical signs to accompany your intuition then go ahead and take a trip to the hospital. They will examine you and will likely ease your fears and send you home. If for some bizarre reason you indeed are unable to feel your contractions then simply count yourself as one of the lucky few. You don't have to feel them for them to be effective, after all, as is proven by women who use epidurals during labor.

Sometimes medical intervention starts labor. When women get closer and closer to their due dates with no sign of labor starting, or when the due date has come and gone, some doctors start bringing up the idea of inducing labor. This is also sometimes used when the mother is experiencing certain problems like pregnancy hypertension or any other condition, which would merit a sooner than later labor. Some doctors will try various methods to jump-start a woman's body into labor. Many doctors wink and suggest a woman go home and have sex with her husband because this is supposed to bring on labor, but really . . . not many women in this condition is looking for some action. Your doctor may suggest stripping your membranes, which is an uncomfortable procedure and many times does not help bring on labor at all. Some of the other techniques are even more drastic and uncomfortable; some doctors utilize a liquid-filled balloon placed in the cervix in an attempt to aid dilation. This procedure is pretty high up on the discomfort scale but it is pretty effective. When these sorts of procedures are unsuccessful in starting up labor some women are induced. This means that various synthetic chemicals are pumped into your body via an IV, bringing on contractions and starting labor.

A word of advice: inducing labor hurts worse than if labor is brought on naturally because the contractions are harder and more painful. Don't look at inducing as a happy and convenient alternative to going into labor naturally. It may appeal to you to pick the day you go in to have the baby, but in the grand scheme of things it is always better to allow nature to take its course.

A C-Section certainly isn't a walk in the park. Sometimes C-Sections are scheduled, and sometimes they are used as a last resort after hours of labor. In some countries it is commonplace to schedule a C-Section from fear of a vaginal labor but it must be remembered that C-Sections, although performed all the time, are major abdominal surgery. The recovery time from a C-Section is longer than with a vaginal delivery, and the baby is more likely to have respiratory problems at birth since the fluid in their lungs isn't squeezed out from pushing through the birth canal. In this sense, you are urged to not think of a C-Section as an easier alternative to birthing your baby, but rather as an alternative method to be used if medically necessary. Having said this, there are times when a C-Section makes sense. Sometimes ultrasounds predict a very large baby, and large babies have a tendency to have problems making their way through the birth canal. Some pregnant women have medical issues which might make the physically demanding aspect of delivering a baby dangerous to their health. There are other women who start the laboring process the natural way and then are eventually told by their doctor that a C-Section is necessary. C-Sections are pretty simple. You're wheeled into the surgery area and are given an epidural or spinal block if you haven't already received one, or some other form of anesthesia. You will lay on your back, most likely with your arms tethered to the sides. A curtain will block your view of the activities, although some hospitals offer mirrors on the ceiling for those moms who want to watch the action. You probably won't feel much pain and will only feel a bit of tugging as the doctors reach in to grab your baby. All in all the process is pretty quick; you will actually spend more time getting sewn back up than you did having the baby pulled out.

It really doesn't matter what method you use to bring your baby into the world as long as both mother and baby are healthy afterwards. You're fortunate to live in a time when you have many option available to you with regards to labor, so it's important to do all the research you can to find the best option for you.

WHAT DOES LABOR FEEL LIKE?

Some pregnant women lose a lot of sleep worrying about what labor is going to feel like. It is no wonder there is such a veil of mystery surrounding labor pains because there really is no way to accurately describe them and interestingly enough many women actually forget what the pain feels like after they give birth. As the old saying goes, if women could accurately remember what going through labor felt like we would be a nation of children with no siblings. So even if you're scared out of your mind over the pain you may experience you can take comfort in the fact that you won't remember the full barrage of pain after it's all over.

NATURAL CHILD BIRTH

It's admirable, but is it necessary? Some women are attracted to the idea of natural child birth because it just seems like the right way to go. Women have been having children without pain assistance for many years, so it seems reasonable enough to many pregnant women that they should be able to do so as well. Other women simply get the heebie jeebies from the idea of having a needle stuck in their back for an epidural and would much rather avoid that scenario. For whatever reason, a woman who is able to endure natural child birth, free of pain medication, should be given some sort of permanent badge to wear that declares to the world that she is amazing.

How does it feel? Labor pains are intense, exhausting, and sometimes feel as though they will go on forever and ever. Yes, there are some women who find labor not to terribly difficult, and yes there are women for whom labor is excruciating. Most women find themselves somewhere in the middle. Contractions feel similar to the worst menstrual cramp ever, multiplied by a hundred. The contractions come in waves, so they start small then build up to an apex of pain before winding back down again. As labor progresses so does the instance of contractions, so some unfortunate women wind up with one contraction after another without any sort of break in between. When the baby crowns many women experience what is dubbed "the ring of fire," which is the burning sensation as the baby's head comes through the vaginal opening. Again, all women are different, and while some women find this to be the most painful part of labor other women say they don't notice it at all.

Be prepared. Women who deliver their babies naturally will often use breathing techniques which don't help so much with the pain but do help the woman focus on the task at hand. If you think you may want to deliver your baby naturally then a good investment would be a birthing class to teach you these sorts of techniques. They will also help you to understand what you're getting yourself into. Another great benefit of taking a birthing class is meeting all the other couples who are in the same situation as you are; some friendships formed in birthing classes last a lifetime!

PAIN MANAGEMENT ASSISTANCE

Plan ahead. Your doctor should go over all the different options for pain management with you well ahead of time. There are some drugs which can be pumped into your body via an IV, but many of these drugs do pass through the placenta and can result in your baby being born a bit drugged up and lethargic. Many women choose these sorts of methods instead of epidurals to avoid the whole needle-in-the-back situation. Whatever method you choose, though, you should alert your doctor of your choice as part of your birthing plan. If you plan on going natural, but there is a small part of you that would like to have the option for some sort of drug if the pain gets too intense, then you need to tell your doctor. If you don't tell your doctor about your intentions you may wind up in labor just as the anesthesiologist has set off on a golfing expedition because he wasn't alerted to be on call.

Is the epidural scary? Sure, it's a little scary. The anesthesiologist will have you sit up and lean forward, probably holding onto the shoulders of your spouse or birthing partner. Then the anesthesiologist stands behind you and puts a really long needle in your back. It's best to just not look, and instead simply concentrate on the imminent pain relief. Sometimes the procedure is pretty painful because anesthesiologists are notorious for not stopping what they're doing even if a really wicked contraction hits, and it's really hard to sit still for a needle in the back when you're in so much pain. After the needle is situated the anesthesiologist will start pumping in the sweet, sweet stuff that either dulls the feelings below the waist or numbs them completely, depending upon the situation. Some women can still feel a bit of what is going on, while other women can't even wiggle their toes.

The case for pain management is a big one. Yes, it would be great to be able to birth a baby without an ounce of pain medication, and many women are able to do just that. The simple fact is that labor is going to be the absolutely most painful experience you have ever had. Couple this with the physical exertion involved plus the emotional aspect as you ready yourself to bring a baby into the world, and the situation simply screams for drugs. You will be able to enjoy the birthing process more if you aren't gnawing on your partner's arm the whole time from the sheer pain of it all. One other perk of pain management drugs that is hardly mentioned is the fact that sometimes there is a need after the birth to do a little stitching, or in some cases to even go in and retrieve the placenta. These activities could be excruciating without some sort of pain medication. Some women prefer to just have that entire area numbed beforehand just in case anything else arises, and this is certainly a valid request.

It's completely normal to be a little apprehensive about what the labor experience is going to be like. Remember that women's experiences vary wildly; some women knit and whistle through their contractions like they are no big deal while other women cry for their mothers and break their husband's fingers. In all likelihood your experience will fall somewhere in between these extremes and you will come through the delivery with flying colors. Your body is a remarkable thing . . . it grew your baby, so it can certainly handle the delivery. When it is all said and done you can be pleased with yourself for how incredibly strong and amazing you are.

WHAT IF . . .

Sometimes things go awry. There is no reason to panic over this fact because the vast majority of deliveries go smoothly and without trouble. For this reason, it is best to not pour over every single problem which may arise and throw yourself into a panic while your brain tries to sort through all the things which can go wrong. Take care of yourself during pregnancy, pick a fantastic medical team for your delivery, and try to relax. Everything will probably go just fine.

DELIVERY ISSUES

Will my husband pass out during the delivery? If you are to believe sitcoms on television then you can rest assured your birthing partner will be splayed out on the floor as soon as labor starts. Fortunately, this doesn't happen in most cases and if it does the medical team is ready. When husbands do pass out during labor it can be for any number of reasons: the sight of blood, the thought of the wife in intense pain, or the combination of these things accompanied by a lack of sleeping or eating or both. It's important that husbands are aware that if they start to feel woozy then really need to tell the medical staff because passing out during labor can entail falling into any number of pieces of medical equipment and this causes a bad situation. Many times if a husband feels the urge to pass out coming on it can be curtailed and avoided with proper techniques, whether it's leaving the room for a breather or sitting down for a minute or two. If your husband does pass out, though, try to cut him some slack. You may not be able to see it all, but labor can be a pretty gory production. For some men, this is just a bit too much to handle.

Do women die in childbirth anymore? Sure, this happens once in a while, but there are usually other medical issues involved and it has become a real rarity in developed countries. The chance of a healthy woman dying from childbirth nowadays is so small that it really isn't something you need to worry yourself about. Honestly, don't you have enough to worry about?

What if I poop/cry/pass out from the pain? Medical staffs in the labor and delivery units have seen it all. Labor, after all, is an incredibly intense process and for many women it can bring out all sorts of interesting behaviors like screaming at their husbands or growling through contractions or sobbing. Try to remember that not only are you going to be in a lot of pain, but also that your hormones are going absolutely bonkers at this point. When you combine a momentous event with intense pain and insane hormones you're bound to see some interesting behaviors. So if you cry, then don't worry about it. Everyone in the room understands that labor hurts and is additionally a very emotional event. Labor isn't an excuse to allow a steady stream of obscenities to flow from your mouth aimed at your hapless husband, though, because remember that although you're in a lot of pain you don't want to emotionally scar your poor husband for life. It certainly is possible to keep your emotions in check to a certain degree when delivering a baby. As far as any sort of bodily functions that you may be worried about, it's important to remember that the medical staff is completely aware of the possibilities of a laboring woman to throw up or pass gas or even to poop while in labor. They are always prepared for these possibilities, and no person in their right mind would ever ridicule a laboring woman for any of these occurrences. Look on the bright side . . . throwing up often helps push the baby further down the birth canal since it engages your abdomen muscles, passing gas may relieve some pressure, and pooping rarely happens but if it does you may not even notice at all. Honestly, there is so much going on down there that poop is the least of your worries.

You'll be hooked up to all sorts of interesting things. Don't be surprised if at some point during labor you take a look around and realize that you are hooked up to all sorts of machines and other odd items. One woman tells of having an IV, a blood pressure cuff, an internal fetal monitor (run through the vaginal opening), and a catheter (also run through the vaginal opening). Having a baby can seem like the most natural thing in the world, but sometimes all the various monitors which are used can make you feel nothing short of a robot. You have the right to have full explanations of each attachment before it is utilized, and in some cases things like IVs are simply routine and may be able to be avoided if you voice strong wishes. Realize, though, that everything is necessary in one way or another, and for now you may need to simply ignore all the various wires and contraptions and concentrate on the labor process.

POST-DELIVERY ISSUES

Even if they have to run additional tests on your baby, he's probably healthy as can be. Many states require that certain tests are conducted on all newborns, so don't be alarmed if your baby has to go through a whole battery of blood tests before you are both discharged. Sometimes your doctor may call in another doctor to get a second opinion on something, like examining the baby's eyes for example. More often than not the second doctor will say that there is no problem, and you should be pleased that your doctor has enough sense to bring someone else in for a peek. If there turns out to be any sort of test results which indicate problems then the medical staff should explain everything fully to you but if you don't understand everything then certainly don't be apprehensive about demanding clarification. You should leave the hospital with a complete understanding of your baby's condition, and if you don't understand then ask more questions until you do.

Sometimes labor results in a significant blood loss. You have probably already realized that due to the nature of what labor is all about there is inevitable blood loss involved. Sometimes, however, the bleeding is excessive or doesn't stop quickly enough. This can be caused by any number of things, such as a placenta, which doesn't detach properly. There are some instances where blood transfusions are necessary, but this is far from the norm. One woman tells of losing a lot of blood during labor but just under the amount required for a blood transfusion. Then, when she was helped to the toilet afterwards by the nurse she started to feel woozy, and promptly passed out while sitting on the toilet. Imagine her surprise when she came to and there she was, still on the toilet with a full staff of medical personnel surrounding her.

Your strength will be shot for a while. Even without significant blood loss, your body has just gone through a tremendously straining event. Don't pick up that suitcase just yet, because you may be surprised at how weak you really are. Your strength will return slowly but surely, but be sure to give your body all the time it needs to return to normal.

You will undoubtedly be plagued at one time or another during your pregnancy by thoughts of all the things, which might go wrong during labor. Take a deep breath and remember that you are having your baby at the most medically advanced time in history. Most labors go smoothly and without major problems. In all likelihood you and your baby will be just fine.

THE HOSPITAL STAY

As strange as it may seem, your hospital stay is probably your best chance to rest up before heading home with your new baby. It's true that being in a hospital room isn't necessarily conducive to relaxing what with the constant monitoring by medical staff and the waves of visitors coming and going from your room. Just try to make the best of the situation and prepare yourself for life with a baby in tow.

VISITORS, FLOWERS, AND SLEEP

Visitors have the best intentions. They show up to ooh and aah over your baby and to hear all about your labor experience. You must make sure of two things, though: make your visitors wash their hands before touching you or the baby, and be firm when it comes to limiting the number of people who visit. Washing hands may seem like a logical thing to do, but many times when someone gets new a newborn all they can think about is holding the little precious bundle. Grandparents are notorious for this sort of behavior. The last thing on their mind is that they may have germs on their hands, but instead they are consumed by the compulsion to hold their new grandchild. Have a bottle of hand sanitizer ready for every single visitor who walks into the room, and don't relent even if Great-Aunt Matilda balks at the notion. The last thing you need right now is to expose your newborn to dirty hands. Along the same lines, try your best to limit the number of visitors you will allow in your room. There will be plenty of time for you and the baby to entertain guests after you head home; right now you need to rest and get to know your baby.

Your hospital room will probably fill up with gifts. If you thought the baby showers resulted in a bunch of baby trinkets and gifts then wait until you see the load you'll get in the hospital room. For whatever reason, people feel obligated to show up with a gift in hand even if they have already presented a gift at a shower. If you don't take care to periodically send these things home with your partner then you may find yourself standing amongst the bounty, scratching your head while trying to figure out how you will get all the things to your car in addition to your bags and the baby. Don't try to balance three vases of fresh flowers while lugging the baby carrier to the car. Just leave the flowers and concentrate on your baby.

It may feel weird, but allow the staff to give you a break. You have waited over nine months for this little bundle of joy to grace your presence, so it may feel like the most unnatural thing in the world to ask a nurse to take the baby to the nursery so you can get some rest. The simple truth, though, is that your baby is probably going to sleep for now, whether he is snuggled up in your arms or if he's swaddled in a blanket at the nursery. The nursery staff is well-trained and will treat your baby with the utmost respect. If your worries revolve around security issues, such as someone tiptoeing into the nursery and stealing your baby, ask your attending nurse about the security measures in place at the hospital. Your nurse will likely put your mind at ease as most hospitals have excellent security methods in place to ensure that everyone in the labor and delivery area is supposed to be there . . . no drifters allowed. Finally, if you feel weird because you worry about things like kidnappers and security measures, don't. This is undoubtedly merely the beginning to a lifetime of worrying about the wellbeing of your child. Just don't let the worries control you and not allow you to enjoy your new baby.

LEARNING ALL YOU CAN

Take it all in now. The nurses and other medical staff who are attending to you and your baby are trained to do just that, so the vast majority of them do it very well. Unless you grew up with younger siblings you may not have the vaguest idea of how to properly bathe a newborn, how to care for the umbilical cord stump, or even how to start breastfeeding. Although you may have wished that the second you laid eyes on your baby that you would magically have all the answers, as though through some divine motherly intuition, for many women the birth of the baby merely helps them to realize that they feel wholly unprepared to care for a newborn. If a nurse suggests something, such as different ways to hold the baby or something else to that effect, take the advice in stride and give it a try. These are seasoned professionals after all, and there really is no harm in trying out their suggestions. If you don't like them, you can always revert back to the old plan of trial and error.

Get involved. Once you feel the strength to do so, get out of bed and get involved with the care of your baby. When the nurse comes in to give the baby its first bath then stand right there assisting. When it's time for a diaper change, grab a diaper and get to work. Now is the best time to learn through trial and error, before you leave the hospital and don't have the benefit of knowing hands there to help you. Don't be passive when it comes to learning how to care for your new baby.

There is no such thing as a stupid question. The medical staff working in the labor and delivery section of a hospital is used to weird questions, and they are trained to answer them without making the mom feel like a complete idiot. In marketing they say that every letter sent to a company is representative of 1,000 opinions, so using this statistic it is logical to assume that any question you ask has either been asked before or has at least been thought of before by some other mom. Babies are born looking a little bizarre sometimes because not only do they have the stress of being squeezed through the birth canal (or surgically removed, which probably isn't too pleasant either) but they also have residuals from mom's hormones to contend with and this makes their appearance a little odd. Babies can be born with enlarged breasts or hair all over their body, or even have cone-shaped heads. It is better to go ahead and ask the questions you may have and go home with the knowledge that everything is okay as opposed to heading home without having asked at all.

Videos, books, and diaper bags, oh my! Some hospitals require new parents to sit down and watch some videos before they are released from the hospital. The typical viewing fare might include a video about general baby care, then another about shaken baby syndrome, and perhaps another about car seat safety. On the one hand the videos are a great idea because they convey such important information, but on the other hand most new parents are exhausted and already confused and this doesn't make for a situation where information is going to be retained very easily. Do your best to take in the information from the videos, but don't hesitate to ask the nurses for clarification if you doze off during the section on ear care. You will probably also be loaded up with books and other freebies from the hospital upon your departure. Any woman who loves getting free samples and other freebies is going to be in Heaven when leaving the hospital. Some moms depart with free diaper bags, formula samples, diaper samples, catalogs, and coupons galore. Go ahead and ask the nurses about what sorts of goodies they have to offer. The samples are usually supplied by companies who want new parents to get familiar with their products, so giving these items away doesn't cost the hospital a cent.

TESTS, RESTING, AND DISCHARGE

You'll both be poked and prodded. Unless you opt for a home birth or a birthing center it is likely that your stay will include periodic checks of you blood pressure and temperature, among other things. These checks are generally taken through the night when you're trying to snooze, and they can get awfully annoying when you're already exhausted. Worse than this, though, is watching the lab technicians come in and do tests on your newborn. Although some hospitals will remove the baby from the room before performing all the necessary blood tests, the majority of hospitals will instead let the lab technician stroll into the room and start poking the baby. If you're already unnerved from the act of labor it can be pretty upsetting to watch the technician stick a small needle in your baby's heel while the baby screams like crazy. Hard as it may seem, just remember that these tests are necessary. The technicians don't like listening to your baby screaming any more than you do, and rest assured that they will not prolong the process any longer than needs be. Also, don't panic if a test comes back with undesirable results. Any test showing something abnormal will likely be repeated in a few days, resulting in better results in most cases. For example, many newborns fail hearing tests in the hospital but then pass a week later because the extra time allows for the fluid to drain from the baby's ears.

Hospital beds may not be so comfortable, but still take advantage of them. Not only are most hospital beds far from comfortable, but also you will probably remain hooked up to an IV for the duration of your stay in addition to whatever else your doctor deems necessary and this can make it downright impossible to find a comfortable spot. Don't be afraid to ask for additional pillows or blankets or whatever you need to feel more comfortable. This is your time to rest up before heading home and dealing with the whirlwind of new parenthood. Try your best to take advantage of the situation.

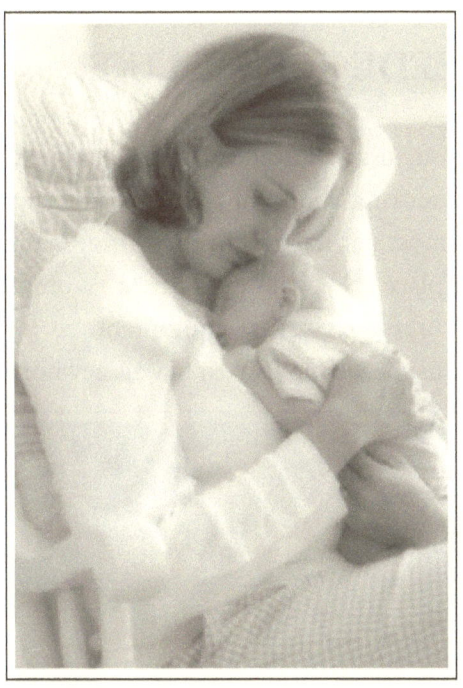

When can you head home with your baby? This depends on a few factors. Some birthing centers allow women to head home with their babies the very same day they go through labor. Most hospitals, however, would like a little bit more time to monitor you and the baby. Vaginal births usually result in being discharged quicker than a Cesarean Section, but sometimes even vaginal births can end up with longer stays. Sometimes mom will get the okay to go home but not the baby, but this situation is always a result of complications and is not the norm. If your delivery was normal, and without any difficulties, then you should be allowed to head home in a day or two. Be sure to let your doctor know if it is your desire to be discharged as soon as possible because some doctors will push tests through and encourage staff to get you out quickly if they know you feel ready to go home. On the other hand, let your doctor know if there is some reason why you don't feel ready to go home. Are you scared to give the baby a bath? Do you not feel physically up to the challenge yet? Let your doctor know your feelings so they can assist you with your concerns.

Your hospital stay is probably going to be a time of mixed emotions. You will want to soak up all the expertise of the medical staff as far as caring for the baby, but at the same time you will be anxious to get home and start your new life as a parent. Try to use your time in the hospital as not only a time to get some rest but also as a time to get to know your wonderful new baby. You may be surprised at just how amazing your baby can be, even when he is just a few minutes old.

WHAT DOES BREASTFEEDING FEEL LIKE?

If your baby looks fragile and weak to you, just wait until you offer your breast and see if you still feel this way. The sucking ability of a baby is amazing. Although breastfeeding is one of the most natural acts in the world, many women can find it a little strange to place their baby to a breast. Women have been taught to consider their breasts as sexual equipment, so for some it seems wholly unnatural and maybe a little icky to have a newborn

sucking on their nipple. With continued feedings, though, the perception of the breast as sexual is replaced with the breast being viewed as functional, life-giving equipment. Heck, before you know it, you may turn into one of those women who whip out their breast in the middle of the mall to feed a baby.

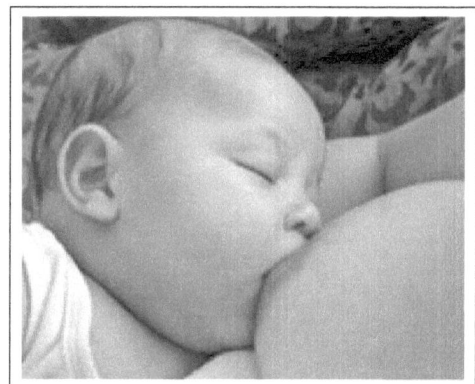

NEVER GIVE UP, NEVER SURRENDER!

Your breasts are about to change BIG TIME. You probably had colostrum to offer your baby when you were in the hospital. Colostrum is the thick white or yellow discharge that comes in either right before you give birth or right afterwards. This offering to your baby is important because it supplies him with antibodies and other things which help him get a great start to being healthy. This isn't your milk though, and if you're like most women you will know exactly when your milk does come in. You may go to bed one night the usual bra size you have always been and then wake up a couple hours later with what appears to be two huge, leaking melons attached to your chest. For many women this can be a painful transition. The very best way to alleviate the pain is to nurse your baby because this will get some of the milk out of your breasts. Luckily, most babies are more than happy to accommodate and if not you can always use a breast pump. You may want to alert your spouse beforehand of this impending change, because men are notorious for seeing these new developments and immediately thinking "va-va-va-voom!" while you're thinking "don't you dare touch these painful things." Investing in a good nursing bra and stocking up on quality nursing pad inserts for your bra will not only provide some comfort but will also prevent accidental milk leaks. One more thing: don't be horrified by your breasts' amazing new ability to squirt milk across the room. It's actually pretty amazing once you get over the initial shock of it.

Yep, it can hurt. It can also be incredibly frustrating. Your baby knows how to suck, but doesn't necessarily understand the intricacies to nursing, and you probably have no idea of what to do other than giving your breast to the baby. Between the two of you, and with the help of a supporting spouse if one exists, you are sure to muddle through and eventually figure it all out. Until then, experiment with several different nursing positions and find the one that works best for you and your baby. Don't assume that just because every picture you have ever seen of a nursing mom has the baby lying across the mom's lap then that must mean that's how it's done. Some babies can't stand this position. Also, give yourself at least a week until you make any sort of decision about giving up with breastfeeding. As long as the baby isn't losing great amounts of weight then you can take this time to work through all the kinks and develop a nursing groove for you and the baby. Your doctor will tell you if it's time to start supplementing with formula, but until then keep on with the nursing. Also be sure to check out all the accessories sold in stores nowadays for nursing mothers. Lanolin ointments can work wonders for tender nipples, and cooling pads are available to slip into your bra between feedings. A word to the wise: discomfort passes quickly, and nursing your baby is unlike anything else in the world. Make a commitment to give it a real try.

Newborns like to eat and eat and eat. Although there aren't any solid statistics out there it is probably likely that mothers who breastfeed get less sleep than mothers who use formula. There are a few reasons for this. Primarily, formula feeding can be done by anyone who can hold a bottle, while nursing moms are pretty much on their own for feedings unless they pump their milk and let someone else feed the baby with a bottle. Secondly, breast milk is digested faster, so while a breastfed baby will likely demand feedings every couple of hours (if not every hour in the beginning), a formula-fed baby will probably be content with feedings stretched out in longer intervals. Realize, however, that the frequent feedings do eventually slow down. Until then it is a good idea to master the art of nursing while resting, either while lying down or while propped up on a comfortable chair.

The benefits of breastfeeding are astronomical. Why should you breastfeed your baby? There are countless reasons, but among them a few stick out. First and foremost are the benefits to the baby. Breastfed babies are generally healthier, have less chance of infections, have higher IQs, and are less likely to be obese later in life. There are also health benefits to the mother. Not only do nursing mothers have a lower incidence of breast cancer later in life, but they also burn up to 500 extra calories daily from nursing which can translate into shedding pregnancy pounds faster. Breastfeeding also forces moms to sit down and rest at regular intervals, which is crucial when recovering from the act of labor. The bonding benefits of breastfeeding are huge; there is nothing quite like knowing that you alone are supplying your baby with nourishment to sustain life. Don't forget also that breastfeeding is free. Purchasing formula can get awfully expensive, and the only cost associated with breastfeeding is keeping the mom fed.

You're going to be hungry. Breastfeeding burns an extra 500 calories a day, which is akin to a serious workout at the gym. You will need to eat more than you would normally, but the trick is to not make the additional calories empty ones. Don't fill up on candy bars and other forms of junk food, but instead eat quality foods to make sure you get enough protein, minerals, and vitamins to keep your milk coming in. One thing some women don't realize is that everything you consume is going to wind up in trace amounts of your milk, and this can have an effect on your baby. If you notice your baby having painful gas every time you have some broccoli then it may be time to nix the broccoli for a while. Some babies are able to handle these things when their digestive system matures a little, while other babies are affected as the months roll by. In some instances, a nursing mom needs to simply avoid certain foods for the duration of breastfeeding. Some babies display severe food allergies, and although breast milk is great to keep their tummy happy the mom may need to follow a strict diet regimen to avoid any allergic reactions on the part of the baby. Some moms will find themselves avoiding any dairy while they nurse due to a baby's lactose intolerance, and this can be particularly difficult for a woman who loves dairy. Remember that breastfeeding never lasts forever (they have to go to college eventually, right?) so right now just consider it taking one for the team.

LACTATION CONSULTANTS

The nature of a lactation consultant can be tricky. Lactation consultants are notorious for forgetting about manners and couth when they approach a new client. They are so used to dealing with their profession that they tend to forget that new moms aren't used to flashing their breasts to everyone who requests to see them. Some lactation consultants will reach right over and squeeze your breast and happily pronounce you as successful in producing colostrum for your baby, and although this is a great development there is still something kind of weird about a complete stranger squeezing liquids from your nipple. Try to realize that this is simply what lactation consultants do for a living, and they are just incredibly passionate about their work. You do have the right, however, to tell a lactation consultant to back off if they make you uncomfortable in any way.

Hospitals sometimes have consultants on staff. During your stay in the hospital a lactation consultant provided by the hospital will probably visit you. This consultant will watch you allow your baby to latch on to your nipple and will ensure that everything is going smoothly. She will probably also go over possible feeding schedules with you in addition to answering any questions you may have. Take advantage of her expertise; although breastfeeding is one of the most natural things in the world it can still be frustrating to a new mom.

You can hire a lactation consultant yourself. After you leave the hospital there are many lactation consultants who will do house calls and help you in any struggles you might be having. Sometimes a new mom will nurse her baby at the hospital without any problems, but then once she gets home and her milk comes in it's a whole new ball game. Lactation consultants can help with positioning issues, feeding issues, and they can even show you how to properly pump your milk. For some women, utilizing the services of a lactation consultant after they leave the hospital can be one of the best services they have ever paid for.

There are breastfeeding organizations you can join. As the old saying goes, "misery loves company." There are times when breastfeeding may seem like misery in the beginning until you work out all the glitches, and sometimes it just feels good to know that you aren't the only mom who is fumbling with nursing. Some breastfeeding organizations are solely about education, while others are social outlets, and still others concentrate on lobbying for breastfeeding legislation. There are some organizations, which do a little bit of all three in addition to other offerings. After you decide what sort of nursing mother you want to be (educated, social, militant, or a mixture of them all) then try seeking out an organization conducive to your needs. You will probably find that the group helps you immensely and you may make some great friends and confidantes whose babies will perhaps later serve as social contacts for your baby.

FORMULA FEEDING

Save this decision for later unless you've already made up your mind. Formula feeding will keep your baby satisfied, but the very best decision for your baby is to breastfeed. It is all too easy to give up breastfeeding in the first few days because it seems too difficult or even to not try breastfeeding

at all. Give yourself the opportunity to attempt breastfeeding, and then if that doesn't work then move ahead with formula feeding. One good tip, though, is to not have formula stocked up in the house when you first arrive home. That makes it all too easy to give up on breastfeeding and head to the pantry to make up a bottle for your baby.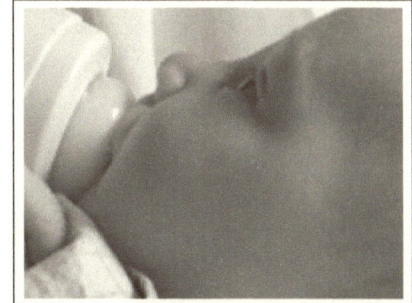

Be sure you understand what you're doing. Some formula comes ready to serve while other formulas need to be diluted or mixed with water. Read the directions every single time you get a new container of formula. Also be sure to familiarize yourself with the sanitary practices involved with formula feedings. Bacteria can breed like wildfire in formula left out of the fridge, especially if your baby has already taken a few sips off the bottle. You'll also have to make sure that every bit of feeding equipment you use is properly sterilized. The last thing you want is to get your baby sick from not cleaning everything like it should be.

Don't beat yourself up over this. If you made an honest effort to breastfeed and found that formula feeding is the way for you then accept the situation and move on. Don't let anyone make you feel inadequate as a mother. Formula fed babies thrive and are healthy too, just like breastfed babies. Shower your baby with love and affection, and they probably won't even notice where the food is coming from.

Whether you breastfeed or formula feed the important thing is that your baby is well fed and satisfied. A well-fed baby is a happy baby. Feeding is much more than helping your baby survive and be healthy, but it is also a great opportunity for bonding. Just wait until you look down while feeding your baby and he looks back into your eyes intently. The love you feel will amaze you.

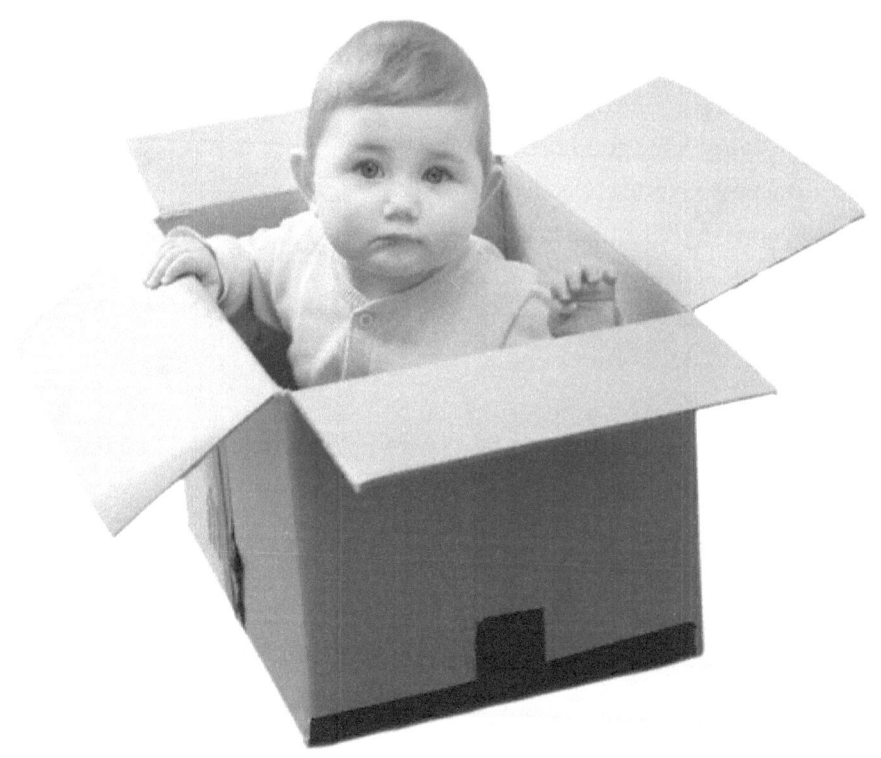

HEADING HOME

Some new parents feel relieved to be released from the hospital because they are ready to start their new life as a family unit. Other new parents feel a little daunted by the task at hand and go home feeling ill prepared for their new roles as parents. All you can do is take everything one day at a time and learn from your mistakes. Besides, it's unlikely your baby will even notice if you don't do things entirely by the book. All your baby wants is to eat, to sleep, and to be adored.

MORE VISITORS, LESS SLEEP

Tell 'em to bring dinner. This is simply not the time for you to be entertaining people. Having a few guests over is great and can be a wonderful pick-me-up, but if you have guests who expect you to play hostess then that's a bad situation. Even if your usual fare includes being an impeccable hostess you need to realize that you're going to be tired from the physical aspects of having a baby and you may actually be a bit cranky from the fatigue and hormonal fluctuations. For this reason, someone who is your best friend in the entire world may become a major annoyance if they hang around the house too long. Guests should come over to fawn over the baby and to help in any way they can. Anyone who comes over for other reasons should wait a while, until you are a bit more settled with your new parental duties.

A message on the answering machine can do wonders. Anyone who has ever had a baby understands that sometimes new parents just need some time to get to know their baby and would rather not entertain guests just yet. Putting a polite yet firm message on your voice mail is a great idea, something akin to "Hi, we're all doing great and getting to know our new Little Blessing. Thanks for calling to check on us, but don't be surprised if we don't get back to you for a while." Anyone who takes offense to such a message probably has never had a newborn to deal with.

Enlist the help of a "New Parents Advocate." If you have a problem with saying no and with asserting yourself then you may want to designate someone else as the Official Bad Guy or Gal. If one of your relatives or friends has come to help out for a while you may want to give him or her specific instructions that you aren't ready for a barrage of visitors. Give your relative the job of minimizing your interruptions, and have them be as firm as needs be. Not only does this help you out tremendously, but you also don't look like the antisocial one.

You know what they say about houseguests and fish. If you live away from your family you will probably receive many offers from relatives who want to come and stay out after the birth of the baby. They come with the premise of being helpful, but sometimes they sort of forget about being helpful and become more of a liability. One sleep-deprived mother had a relative come to visit shortly after the birth of her son and the relative indulged in luxurious naps on the couch often while the new mom stumbled around in a sleep-deprived stupor. Another new mom tells of a mother-in-law who came to stay after the birth of her first-born. The mother-in-law never offered to help, refused to change diapers, and spent a great deal of time complaining about her daughter-in-law's hormonal swings. Unfortunately, a situation like this truly degrades the new parents' experience and makes it even harder to get into the groove of caring for a newborn. Before accepting a relative or friend's offer to come visit after the baby is born think long and hard about what sort of effect the person is likely to have. It is also best to limit the time a houseguest stays. Some hosts can handle two weeks worth of visitors while others can barely tolerate a three day visit.

On the other hand, some people love having visitors. Not everyone needs to regulate the amount and duration of visits from well-wishers. There are some people who relish the attention and who also are blessed to have visitors who truly want to help. One new mom looks back fondly on when her relatives came to visit. The relatives cleaned, cooked, filled the house with groceries, and insisted on taking the baby once in a while so the new mom could get some much needed rest. So don't feel odd if you would rather have a house full of visitors after the birth of your baby, just be sure you know what you're getting yourself into . . . and make sure they all wash their hands!

BIG CHANGES

Are you going to stay home with the baby? Many new moms have the double whammy of trying to figure out how to deal with a new baby while also taking on the new role of a stay-at-home mom. For many women the idea of not bringing in a paycheck can really take some getting used to. Many of these women are also overwhelmed by the idea of being solely responsible for the upkeep of the house in many instances whereas the chores were previously divided between her and her husband (albeit unevenly, if statistics are true). Don't be surprised if one day you look around at your house in a messy state of shambles, no dinner on the table, your husband walking through the door and you're still in your pajamas. These instances happen to more new moms than they care to admit, and if you can keep your sense of humor intact about everything then you are much less likely to allow situations like this to upset you. Just know that it is going to take you a little while to get to a point where you can efficiently handle everything and embrace your role as a stay-at-home mom. There will come a time where you actually find that you have some extra time on your hands, and this is one of the great advantages of being a stay-at-home mom; you can take online college classes, start up a small home business, or think about having another baby (more on that later).

Are you returning to work? There are many different reasons why some moms decide to return to work. For some women it's simply a financial necessity. Other women aren't willing to give up their careers, and still other women say that they would like their babies to be exposed to other babies in day care on a daily basis. The decision to stay home or return to work is a decision which every woman must make, and the right decision is simply whichever scenario is best for you. If you know that you intend on returning to work and you don't have a spouse who can stay home with the baby then it is imperative to start the search for a great daycare provider while you are still pregnant. In some cities there is a real lack of quality day care providers so it is important to conduct a thorough search and have a spot reserved before you even give birth. There are a couple of different routes you can check out. Some people prefer large day care centers while other people prefer a home-based day care.

Some parents are fortunate enough to have trusted relatives or friends who can take the baby during work hours, and some parents decide on a live-in nanny. You have many options to choose from, but the important thing is to make sure you do plenty of research and come up with a daycare plan which makes you, your spouse, and your baby comfortable. Realize that the first few times you drop your baby off at day care you will probably sob worse than the baby, just make sure to save the tears until you get into the car otherwise you're sending the message to your baby that it's a bad situation.

Don't let your relationship with your spouse deteriorate. As hard as it is to fathom right now, there will come a time when your baby and subsequent children will leave the home and you will be right back where you started: you and your spouse in an empty house. If you spend the next eighteen or so years putting your entire focus on your children and not your spouse then you may look at each other years down the road and not know a thing about each other except your parenting styles. Yes, it is extremely difficult to worry about your spouse when your baby is demanding so much of your time and attention, and you may be in a situation where you feel disjointed since you either can't indulge in intimate time because you haven't received the okay from your doctor or you're just too darn tired. There are other ways to feel connected to your spouse, and sometimes a quick, "Hey, do you know that I adore you?" will do wonders when you're in the middle of helping each other clean up a bad diaper incident. Don't forget what made you fall in love with your spouse to begin with.

EXHAUSTION AT ITS BEST

Sleep when your baby sleeps. You will hear this time and again, and you will probably immediately think of all the things you need to get done while the baby sleeps: laundry, e-mails, the dishes, or whatever. The quicker you learn to sleep when your baby sleeps, the better. It's amazing what a quick twenty minute nap will do for a tired mom. Right now your main concern should be building your strength back up and taking care of your new baby, not checking off items on a to-do list. Get into the habit of laying down right after you put your baby down for a nap, and keep this pattern until you begin to feel a little less like a zombie and a little more like your old self.

Don't leap up at the first peep your baby makes while sleeping. This advice is especially hard for new parents to follow because of the fear that their newborn will stop breathing in the middle of a nap or when asleep at night. Some parents also feel obligated to comfort their newborn at the first sign of discomfort. For these reasons new parents often feel compelled to rush to check on the baby if he cries or gurgles or otherwise sounds like he may be waking up. The truth of the matter is that if babies are left to their own devices they will often settle down and fall back asleep on their own. Sometimes going in and checking on the baby is enough distraction to wake the baby up fully, thereby unintentionally ending the nap. For some parents, it is helpful to keep a watch nearby and time the duration of the baby's stirring. Having a set time such as thirty seconds or a minute where you allow the baby to stir and gurgle until he decides if he wants to wake up or not might be helpful. If, however, the idea of not rushing to your baby's aid the second he makes a sound seems uncomfortable to you then don't force it. Of all the advice you receive regarding your baby the very best advice is to trust your gut instinct. Don't do anything which feels wrong. If you want to sleep on the floor next to the crib just to make sure the baby is breathing then go ahead. Chances are, though, that this will get old fast.

Have you considered co-sleeping? Experts go back and forth about the idea of co-sleeping, and currently the trend appears to be against it. Many women fall into co-sleeping without ever intending to do it; maybe in a heap of exhaustion they lay their screaming baby down on the bed and then lay down next to him, only to find the baby is suddenly content lying next to mommy. Or for other women they master the laying position for nursing and accidentally doze off only to wake up with the baby, still attached, snoozing right next to her. Still other women plan to co-sleep before the baby is even born. Either way, it's worth taking a look at. Co-sleeping is not a new trend; it has been around for thousands of years and is still the norm in some countries today. Babies like co-sleeping because they are close to mom, and moms like co-sleeping because they are close to baby and they usually find that their babies sleep better than they would in a crib. Co-sleeping is not all sunshine and roses though as there are many precautions that parents need to take to lower the risk of the baby suffocating in the bed. That means no fluffy pillows, no fancy comforters, and really no deep sleep for either parent. Some parents don't like the idea of giving up their intimate time with their spouse due to a baby in the bed with them. It is also pretty hard for some parents and their babies to make the transition from co-sleeping to the crib since the baby has only ever slept with mom and dad and isn't used to sleeping alone. This issue should be discussed with your partner if you're considering it because if both parents aren't on the same page about co-sleeping then it can lead to resentment. If you do decide on co-sleeping, though, you will probably find that some of your favorite memories of your baby have to do with him nestling up next to you for a good night's sleep.

ACCEPT HELP!

The last thing you need to worry about is cleaning your house. Here is a secret that you might as well know about now: after your baby is born, your laundry will probably never be all done ever again. Your sink may remain free of dishes for a short while, but in all likelihood this condition is temporary. Let's not even get started talking about what your bathrooms will look like. Yes, there is something to be said about a nice, tidy house and yes, you don't want to allow your house to fall into the status of a health hazard. For right now, though, the important thing is to get rest and get to know your baby. The house will start to get back into shape after you figure out some tricks, like putting the baby in a front carrier while you vacuum or singing to your baby while you do the dishes. Don't worry about these things in the first few weeks after your baby is born. You can bet that you will be able to spend more time worrying about dust and dirt on the floor once your baby starts putting everything in his mouth and crawling.

Take-out menus are a beautiful thing. Unless you had the foresight to bake and freeze dozens of casseroles, or even better if your spouse is a willing and able chef, then you will probably be ordering out for a good portion of your meals after you bring the baby home. In some communities it is customary for neighbors, friends, and relatives to bring over meals to new parents, but if you don't have this sort of social advantage then you will be on your own. Even if you generally enjoy cooking there will be some nights when you will be simply too tired to attempt a home cooked meal. Try to get to know which restaurants around your town deliver, and try your best to pick healthy meals. Having a newborn and being exhausted are not justification for eating a triple cheeseburger and French fries every night.

The moral of the story is that you need to take this time to rest, get to know your baby, and not fret about chores and other things, which can surely wait a little while until you're ready to tackle them. Trust your instincts and don't allow other people to tell you what to do if their ideas are contrary to what feels right for you. Your grandmother may indeed be a wise woman, but remember that when she had babies they put babies to sleep on their stomachs and made sure babies received sunbaths daily. Times do change, and when your baby someday grows up and has babies of his own he will probably scoff at your advice too. That's just the way it goes.

WHAT YOUR BABY CAN DO

LEARNING, LEARNING, LEARNING!

Your baby is a mini-scientist. Scientists form theories and test them, and this is exactly what babies do. Your baby's theory may be as simple as "if something is put in my mouth and I suck on it then milk comes out sometimes" to as complex as "if I cry then mommy fixes whatever the problem is." This scientist mentality only gets stronger as your baby gets older, and by the time your baby reaches toddler hood you will be amazed at how such profound thoughts can come from such a little person.

You are your baby's favorite subject. You can put all the flashcards or primary colored pictures in front of your baby as you want, but nothing will compare to your face when it comes to your baby's preference for something to look at. Babies have an innate desire to seek out faces, and from the very beginning your baby is busy trying to learn the intricacies of your facial structure. Researchers have even mapped out how babies gaze at a mom or dad's face in a certain repeatable pattern. That's how serious your baby is about getting to know the contours of your face. Be sure to allow your baby plenty of time to simply study your face. For babies, it's the most beautiful thing they have ever seen.

Enjoy seeing the world through the eyes of a newborn. For the first couple of weeks a newborn doesn't seem to notice much. They spend a lot of time dozing and eating without much regard for the world around them. The suddenly their eyes open wider than ever and they are interested in everything around them. You will be able to tell what interests him by studying his body language and listening to the noises he makes. One of the biggest perks of being a parent is being able to see the world through your children's eyes. You may have seen a cat every day for your entire life, but when you introduce your baby to a cat for the first time your baby's excitement will be infectious. You'll notice all the cool things about cats that you hadn't really noticed in a long time. Now is the time to explore new places with your baby: zoos, gardens, art museums, and even a plain old shopping mall are great locations to explore with your baby.

SLEEPING, POOPING, AND EATING

Babies do like to sleep, just in short increments. If you envisioned your baby taking regularly scheduled naps and then sleeping through the night then you are probably in for a big disappointment. Although it is true that some babies are good sleepers, taking to sleeping through the night early on and eagerly accepting nap time as a time of rest, the vast majority of babies have no idea that night time signifies sleep time and that nap time is not the time to fill their diapers with a gift for mom. Babies simply need to be taught to sleep in regular intervals, and this takes time and effort. Until then, don't be shocked if your baby has a sleep/wake cycle which seems erratic and unpredictable. Rest assured that eventually your baby will ease into a schedule, probably consisting of a morning nap, an afternoon nap, and then a full night's sleep. This glorious development, however, will take some time. Be patient.

That's not tar coming out of your baby. The first few poops that a baby has can be downright scary for new parents if they aren't expecting the dark, sticky substance of which first poops consist of. This is temporary, and it's actually your baby pooping out amniotic fluid. This stuff is so sticky that you may find you need to use a ton of wipes to remove it all from your baby's behind. Don't fret; this tar-like pooping only lasts a couple of days and then it will be on to more recognizable bowel movements which, although pretty gross at times, at least do not resemble sticky motor oil.

The only thing a baby likes more than sleeping is eating. Parents are often cautioned to not utilize feeding as a means to calm down an infant too much, and the reason why they are cautioned about this is because it works so darn well! Upset babies are magically transformed into happy babies when a nipple or bottle is stuck in their mouth. This is because not only do babies like eating, but the act of sucking calms them immensely. Make sure your baby is well fed and don't beat yourself up too much if you occasionally use feeding as a means to comfort and calm your baby. Just don't make it your usual fare, because you need to learn how to comfort your baby in other ways or you will likely wind up with one chubby baby.

EMOTIONAL ATTACHMENT AND BONDING

It's okay if it's not love at first sight. Many times new parents will expect to immediately fall in love with their new baby only to realize when the baby is born that they don't feel instant warm feelings. For some parents it's the initial shock of seeing a baby emerge from the mom . . . intellectually they knew there was a baby in there but sometimes nothing can really prepare a mom for seeing another human being come out of her and for dads it can be weird to see a baby pop out of a place which was normally reserved for intimacy. If that shock isn't enough, add to the mix a good dose of exhaustion after a hard labor experience or a draining Cesarean Section and a hormonal surge and this may equate to a less than magical moment when a parent meets a new baby. There is no need to feel guilty if you aren't immediately smitten with your newborn, and in almost all cases the feelings of immense adoration will come soon enough. It won't be long before you're standing over your baby's crib, staring intently at your baby and crying over how much you love him.

Your protective impulses may surprise you. You will probably have to train yourself to not think that every man in the store is a kidnapper, that not every corner is a route to a band of gypsies whose main goal is to steal babies, and that not every little old lady who stops to fawn over your baby is trying to figure out a way to wrestle your baby from your arms. Truly, the protective impulses you will experience will sometimes be so strong that you will even surprise yourself in your thinking. This is nature's way of insuring that you watch out for your offspring; you just need to keep in check so that you have a healthy dose of paranoia instead of a debilitating dose which keeps you from leaving the house. If all else fails, keep muttering "not everyone is out to steal my baby" to yourself while you are out and about until you actually believe it.

Your baby adores you like no other. Although newborns are not yet to the stage where they can display any real separation anxiety they still have a preference for their parents, more specifically, for their mothers. There is a bond between newborns and their moms which was in the making the entire time the mom was pregnant. Newborns prefer the sound of their mother's voice and many will actually turn towards their mother when they hear her speaking. Newborn babies know their mom's scent, and magically find just the right way to nestle into their mom's arms. Enjoy this time of Mommy Worship from your baby since it certainly won't last forever.

Quite simply, your baby is amazing. His brain is working overtime to try to make sense of the world around him while he continues to dazzle you with his perfection. This is the time to learn all you can about your baby and to start to teach him about his surrounding environment. The most important thing for your baby right now is for you to make sure he feels safe and loved.

AFTER THE DUST CLEARS

Do you feel like running to the store on the corner to get a bag of chips? This simple jaunt used to be a quick errand that didn't really require much planning. Now, with a newborn, you may find yourself paralyzed with fear that taking your baby out will result in the baby getting exposed to germs, or kidnapped, or abducted by aliens, or whatever your chosen paranoia may be regarding going out. The truth of the matter is that newborns are highly portable, and once your doctor gives the okay to take your baby on outings you'll soon realize that it just takes some getting used to. The same goes for all other aspects of your life with a newborn: *it just takes some getting used to.*

LIFESTYLE CHANGES

You're not #1 anymore. It doesn't really matter anymore what your temperature preference is in the house; if your baby isn't comfortable then you need to adjust it. It doesn't matter that the playoff games are on TV; if the television proves too be too much stimulation for your baby then it needs to be shut off. You're no longer living only for you, or even for your spouse. Your main priority is your baby, and that's the way it should be. No more late nights out and no more wasting money on unnecessary purchases, it's time to grow up and be a parent. Your baby is counting on you to make the right decisions. Yes, a time will come when you can focus a little more on yourself, but for right now your baby is number one.

It's hard to schedule appointments when you never know when you might get pooped on. At some point your baby will work himself into a sleeping schedule which will allow you to make appointments at a pretty predictable pace, but until then you will be happy to discover that most newborns are pretty portable if they are in a carrier. This allows for you to transfer the baby from the car without waking him up, consequently allowing you to get your shopping done or attend a doctor's appointment or whatever it is you need to get done. The major thing to take into consideration, though, is that babies have a tendency to have exploding diapers or major spit-up episodes at the most inopportune time. You may be heading into church service and realize that your baby has had a major bowel movement which has seeped out of his diaper and down your shirt. The old motto of "be prepared" is very appropriate here. Even though you may already be feeling a bit like a pack mule with the diaper bag you may want to consider throwing a change of shirt in there for you too. At the very least, keep a spare shirt in the car. You never know when you might need it.

You may notice a big priority change. Maybe you always made sure to schedule a weekly manicure, or perhaps your favorite pastime on a Sunday morning was to lazily read the newspaper while sipping hot tea. These things may not become any less appealing to you, but for now these indulgences may need to go on the backburner. Don't worry; you will eventually get your beloved Sunday paper ritual back, but right now is the time to revel in your baby because believe it or not he is going to grow up very quickly right before your very eyes.

Occasionally pull yourself away from the baby for a breather. Many new moms have the distinct problem of desperately wanting a moment or two to themselves but not entirely trusting anyone else to take care of the baby, even their spouse. You really need to take some time to catch your breath and be something other than a walking spit-up sponge. Even if your partner does things completely different than you do you need to realize that sometimes different can be good. Your spouse may actually take it as an insult if you don't allow him time alone with the baby because that sends a signal that you find him inept. Make a concerted effort to get out once in a while, even if it is a quick dash to the grocery store. The brief experience will refresh you and ultimately make you a happier mom. Remember, if you have a competent and loving spouse there is absolutely no reason why you should have to deal with your baby twenty-four hours a day, seven days a week, all by yourself.

POSTPARTUM DEPRESSION

Hormones can be a bummer. Every new mom goes through a hormone surge after delivering a baby, but the extent of the surge is what makes some women ecstatic while others are unbearable. Some women have a predisposition towards postpartum depression if they had previously dealt with depression. When is it "baby blues," and when is it depression? Baby blues is a result of hormones and the other factors which all form together to make a new mom feel a little sad and overwhelmed. Postpartum depression can either be an extension of baby blues or an entirely different beast. If you feel as though you're in a funk and you feel a little like crying sometimes then it's probably just a dose of baby blues and will clear up as your hormones regulate themselves.

No sleep + hormones = crankiness. You're about to find out how strong you really are. Not only will you give birth to a baby but then you will attempt to recover while also caring for your new baby while not getting anywhere near the amount of consistent sleep you're supposed to. This can be a Herculean task indeed. It's no wonder that many women find themselves a bit moody at times. If you find yourself poising to snap at your husband about what a miserable bum he is then it's probably time to take a breather. As you find yourself getting a little more sleep and as your hormones start to regulate themselves a little better than you will surely find yourself in a better mood. If you find your emotions often fly off handle no matter how much you try to keep them in check then be generous with sincere apologies to whoever received the brunt of your wrath whether it's your husband, the mailman, your mother, or whoever else rubbed you the wrong way.

There comes a time when you should seek help. So-called "baby blues" can turn ugly, and there is a time when you simply can't handle these feelings by yourself anymore. If you ever get the feeling that you can't go on, or if you find yourself harboring feelings of wanting to hurt yourself or your baby, then you need to contact your doctor immediately. If the feelings grip you while you are alone with your baby and you can't shake the feelings then you need to contact anyone who can come take your baby from you so you can get a breather and make sure your baby is safe. It may seem like a totally foreign concept that some women feel as though they might hurt their babies, but postpartum depression can do bizarre things to a woman's thinking patterns. There is help for this condition, including psychotherapy, exercise, and medication. Your doctor is the very best resource for questions regarding postpartum depression.

Friends are a depression-buster. Try seeking out other women who are in a similar situation as yours. There are support groups for new moms all over the place, and a quick internet search will find a group suitable to you. Sure, your spouse can listen to you and offer support, but sometimes there are some things which only a new mom can understand and sympathize with. A common trend is for new moms to either intentionally or unintentionally distance themselves from their friends who don't have children, and this sometimes can leave these new moms without a social outlet. The good news is that a baby is the best conversation starter among new moms, and your newest pal might be a woman you meet at the mall who has a similar stroller.

FINANCIAL CONCERNS

Diapers aren't cheap. If you are planning on using disposable diapers one of the very first things you will notice is how incredibly expensive they can be, especially in the first few months when your baby is a veritable pooping machine. You can try cloth diapers, but often these are simply not as portable as disposables. Some women use cloth diapers at home and then disposables when out and about, and this seems like a good plan. If you are using disposables then accept this little bit of advice: you don't need to buy the most expensive diapers as the less expensive diapers work just as well. Generic and store brands, however, are a different story. These kinds of diapers are cheap for a reason . . . they leak more and simply aren't as comfortable for your baby. So buy the less-expensive brand name diapers and by all means utilize coupons. An insider's tip: you can call diaper manufacturers to get on their mailing list and they will keep you well stocked in coupons mailed directly to your house.

One income instead of two incomes can be a shocker. If you decide to stay home with your new baby for some time instead of immediately returning to work you may be shocked at the drop in income. Before you give birth, when you are making the decision of if you should stay home, you and your spouse need to sit down and figure out a realistic budget with only one income. Some financial experts suggest that you should try to live with the one income a few months prior to your baby being born and stash the second income into a savings account. This serves as not only a great primer for surviving with one income but it also builds up a nice chunk of change for the savings account as a safety umbrella after the baby comes. If you find that you are constantly going into the red each month then it's time for a budget revision. Many people have the income to eliminate one source of income, but it takes meticulous budgeting and giving up certain non-essentials. Really though, isn't it worth it to give up those daily designer coffees in order to stay home with your baby?

Hand-me-downs can be great. Some parents can go for months without having to buy a single piece of clothing for their baby because they are lucky enough to have a friend or relative who happens to have a nice stash of clothing from a previous baby. If you are offered hand-me-downs from someone think twice before turning them down. You never know what sort of great clothes may be in store for you. Remember that babies grow out of clothes relatively quickly, so a bag of hand-me-downs may include some pieces which have either been worn only once or twice or even some pieces of clothing which still have price tags attached. What some hand-me-down recipients do is immediately divide the clothing they receive into two piles: one pile for the clothing they like and another pile for the clothing which is either too stained or just not their style. The clothing you don't like can go to charity, and the person who gave you the clothes doesn't need to know that you didn't utilize all the clothing. Be sure to compose a nice thank you note too, because although second hand clothing isn't bought in the store it is still a really nice gesture.

Babies don't need designer clothes. It is really easy to get tempted by some of the designer baby clothing stores in the mall. The clothes they make are so incredibly cute! It is difficult to not go on a shopping spree and then justify it by simply wanting the best for your baby. There are times when fancy outfits are considered justifiable, like for portraits, but they don't necessarily need to break the bank. Baby clothes should be functional first and foremost, and leave it to your baby to make the clothes look adorable. Your money is better spent in other ways.

Start a college fund right now. Speaking of better ways to spend your money, consider starting a college fund immediately after your baby is born. Even if you only contribute a small amount like $20 a month it will certainly add up to a respectable amount by the time your child is ready to start college. That is, of course, unless your baby is a prodigy and will start college at 13, but then surely there will be scholarships galore available. The point is that small contributions coupled with compound interest will make for a nice college account. Be sure to talk to your bank about the various accounts available; there are some tax-deferred accounts which are a much better product for this particular instance than a regular savings account would be. Try having the monthly amount automatically withdrawn from your account every month so you don't miss a month.

Don't go nuts. Do you really need a new minivan after your baby arrives? Your baby will be just as happy in the backseat of your old sedan as long as he is securely strapped into a car seat. You will probably notice an intense urge to upgrade almost everything in your life after the baby is born since you simply want the best for him. Don't burden yourself with new bills. All a new baby needs is sleep, food, and love. He couldn't care less what the drapes look like.

Once you get home with your new baby the real fun begins. If you can get past the sleeplessness and utter confusion which accompanies the new parent experience then you will quickly realize that your newborn is simply amazing. The lifestyle changes you have to make pale in comparison to the sheer joy you'll feel when your baby looks up at your and grants you a beaming smile.

TIME TO TEACH

Unless your baby is enrolled in some sort of daycare program, you are the person who is primarily responsible for teaching your baby about the world around him. Babies aren't passive for very long; they yearn to figure out the world around them and will do well if they have an active and enthusiastic teacher who is willing to expose them to new things and teach them the fine art of play. You don't need fancy books and expensive classes to raise a smart kid, although these things can be a lot of fun.

BABY CLASSES

Marketing starts young nowadays. You may be surprised to hear that some parents start their babies in classes as young as four weeks old, but it's true. There are many play classes which claim to enhance a baby's learning and teach valuable social skills at a very young age. The truth of the matter is that although some babies will indeed enjoy the vibrant colors and the fun music, for other babies it can be downright overwhelming. Does this mean that parents should steer clear of enrolling their babies into these sorts of classes? No, not necessarily. There are pros and cons to baby classes. Some of the cons include exposure to germs, sometimes ridiculous tuition costs, and over stimulation to sensitive babies. The pros, however, are numerous as well. There are some babies who get a real kick out of the classes, but the real benefit is truly to the new parent. Where else can you take your baby and chat with other parents who are just as confused as you are as to what you're supposed to be doing when raising a newborn? Classes like these can be superb social outlets for parents, and in some cases lifelong friendships can be formed. One woman tells of a baby class she joined when her daughter was seven weeks old. She instantly connected with some of the other moms and they formed a playgroup outside of the class. Now as the children of the playgroup are all nearing age three the moms are pleased to see them have these relationships with other little girls who they have known for practically their whole young lives. Many of the moms from this playgroup still attend play classes with their daughters because they feel the classes help with their daughters' cognitive and social development. The moral of the story is this: if you're willing to pay the costs for the classes and you aren't expecting the classes to turn your child into some sort of genius, then go for it. Sometimes it's a big relief to get to talk to someone in the same boat.

Is your baby a gymnast? As if play classes weren't enough, some children centers offer gymnastic classes for babies as young as three months old. Although it's true that a three month old is not likely to master the high bar at this age, these sorts of classes stress physical development and often tout themselves as being tiered programs designed to develop children into eventual gymnasts. As the children get older they move up to more advanced classes involving actual gymnastic moves, but in the beginning the classes are mostly designed to get your baby moving. As with the aforementioned play classes it is best to not have unrealistic goals in mind when enrolling your baby into these sorts of classes. Your baby is probably not going to be the next gold medalist on the Olympic gymnastics team. If you do enroll your baby in a gymnastics class, be sure that you're doing it for social interaction and so your baby can have some fun. Any other reason is doomed to eventually backfire.

Talk to your baby sooner. One of the most frustrating things about taking care of a baby is that sometimes you simply can't figure out what the baby wants. They cry and scream and thrash about and you know there is something they are desperately longing for. The fact that you can't figure out what it is makes you feel completely inadequate as a parent and in turn frustrates the heck out of you, making your baby even more frustrated. Sign language classes to the rescue! At around six months of age you can enroll your baby into a sign language class that is designed to teach both you and the baby signs for vital words like milk, juice, and food. The concept behind the class is to allow your baby to convey to you their needs much sooner than if you were to wait for them to open their mouths and say, "milk please, dearest mother." Do sign language classes work? It really depends on the baby, but for the most part it is truly possible to teach a baby a few simple signs to make things a little easier. Do you need a class to teach you this? Not really. There are countless books on the subject which can teach you just as well, so if you're signing up for a class you should do it either for the social aspect or because you simply prefer a class setting rather than trying to go it alone with advice from a book. Some studies have shown, however, that a number of babies who are taught to sign actually take a little longer to start speaking. This makes sense in theory since there's no reason to talk when they have alternate means to communicate.

Interactive exercise classes can be great. Some places offer exercise classes geared towards new moms which allow you to bring your baby with you and in some cases actually let your baby join you in the fun. This can be a lot of fun for both you and your baby, and will also help you get back into your pre-pregnancy jeans a little faster. These classes can also be a great social outlet, and you're teaching your baby from a very young age that physical exercise can be fun. Check with your local gym to see if they offer baby exercise or yoga classes.

Don't over schedule your baby. You may think that the more classes the better for your baby's intellectual and social development, but the truth is that babies, particularly newborns, can get over stimulated quite quickly. Take the cue from your baby; if he starts fussing and crying during the class then remove him from the situation and sit somewhere quietly with him to see if that calms him down. Realize too that swim classes, which are popular for newborns, may not be the best idea either since this exposes your baby's delicate skin to chlorine and other chemicals. Besides, does a six week old really need to know how to swim?

READING

Your baby loves the sound of your voice. It really doesn't matter if you aren't the best reader. Your baby is in love with your voice, so it's important to regale your baby with some reading every day. It doesn't even have to be a silly baby book, but you can read to your baby whatever it is you're reading at the time: the business section of the newspaper, assembly directions for a new toy, the ingredient listing on the side of the cereal box. Read to your baby often and passionately, and you will likely have a baby who will embrace reading in the future with great vigor.

Books help your baby's brain. Books aren't all about the baby listening to the melodic sound of your voice. The repetition of stories and the chance to listen to speech makes for great brain building. When you read to your baby, little neurons within your baby's brain are busily making connections and teaching your baby all about the surrounding world. If you want to actively participate in building your baby's brain power then you should read to them every single day.

Reading makes for good bonding. Reading is something which should be shared between a parent and baby quite often. The physical act of reading, with the snuggling on the lap and the frequent hugs and squeezes, helps remind the baby that they are loved and cared for. The ritual behind reading becomes a familiar practice for the baby, and babies love and crave familiarity. Reading simply makes for a great bonding opportunity between you and your child, so crack open a book and get reading!

THE TELEVISION DEBATE

Babies need to move, learn, and interact. You can buy all the educational movies and TV shows that you want to, but the simple fact of the matter is that babies learn best by moving and exploring the world around them. Watching television is an extremely passive pastime, and at this stage in your baby's development a video simply cannot offer the same learning potential as play can. Young babies will probably learn more about the world around them by simply staring into their mother's eyes as opposed to being plucked down in front of the television to watch a show. Also remember that what you do with your baby now is setting the stage for future habits . . . if the idea of a teenager who won't get off the couch because they're watching television makes you shudder then take care to not send the message to your baby that TV is a fantastic entertainment medium.

Baby brains don't understand that TV shows are fictional. You have probably noticed by now that even very young babies can easily pick up on the emotions of the people around them. If you cry, your baby is likely to start crying too. It's not that your baby is upset about the same thing you are upset about, but rather that your mood affects their mood. Imagine, then, a young baby exposed to a trashy daytime talk show, complete with paternity tests and flying chairs. If everyone on the TV screen is screaming at each other and throwing punches your poor baby will simply not understand what in the world is going on. If you insist on having the television on then it's best to censor what your baby is exposed to.

A mommy has to do what a mommy has to do. Having said all this, there are simply some times when a mommy needs to take a break. Honestly, not every woman can be in animated Mommy Mode all day long, and sometimes chores looming or sheer exhaustion simply takes over. Some moms have the best intentions when they declare that their children will never watch television, but these same women often eventually turn to TV in moments when they simply need a break from their kids. This is completely understandable, and a parent shouldn't beat themselves up over an occasional bending of the "no television" rule. The key is to try to not use the TV as a babysitter, but instead try to stay in the room, commenting on what the child is watching and remaining vigilant so they don't wind up watching something inappropriate. Don't let the television take over the day's activities either; you may be surprised to find that your baby will sit for quite some time in front of the television without protest. Try to limit the viewing time to short intervals, perhaps thirty minutes. It's amazing what a nice thirty minute break from serenading your baby with "Itsy Bitsy Spider" will do for a parent's attitude.

You are the primary teacher for your baby's first few years of life. You need to decide what sort of teacher you want to be, and have a game plan. You will learn early on what method your baby prefers, whether they want you to be active and boisterous or instead passive and deliberate. The best advice to new parents when it comes to helping their babies learn is to think of every moment as a teaching moment. The leaves on the lawn which used to be annoyances are now science lessons. The smooth bedspread is a lesson in tactile learning. An unexpected breeze is a lesson in climate changes. Try not to get caught up in the hustle and bustle of carting a baby to and fro, and instead realize that your baby is primed for learning . . . all you need to do is supply the lessons.

READY FOR ANOTHER ONE?

Nature has a strange way of allowing women to forget about the pain of childbirth so that they will eventually start wanting to got through the whole process again. Some researchers have said that there is a chemical, which is released into woman's body shortly after giving birth which actually erases some of the memories of intense pain associated with contractions and birth. No wonder some women are ready to jump back in and have another baby pretty quickly. You need to take several factors into consideration before taking the leap again because having another baby is going to change things a lot . . . in some cases more than having the first baby did.

HOW LONG TO WAIT

Are you physically ready? Maybe it has always been your intention to have your children close in age and you're ready to try to get pregnant again very quickly after having your first baby. You need to take into account the physical strain that pregnancy has on your body. Think about it; your body played host to a growing human for nine months. That takes a toll on a body, and you need time to recover. You should also do your very best to lose the weight you gained with your first pregnancy before getting pregnant again. This may seem incredibly counterproductive since you know you'll pack on the pregnancy pounds again, but you may find that you simply don't lose weight as easily after the second pregnancy, especially if the pregnancies were close together. This doesn't hold true for all women, but it is more often than not the case. The best thing you can do is talk to your doctor before attempting to conceive. The doctor will probably do some tests to make sure your protein levels are up and your iron levels are fine and whatever else your doctor deems necessary. Once you get the thumbs up from your doctor then you're ready to go. By the way, it is entirely possible to conceive a baby when you're breastfeeding, contrary to popular belief that nursing has a fail-safe contraceptive effect. Some women even choose to continue nursing through the pregnancy, and there are some women who have the strength to nurse both their toddler and newborn in tandem. Now that's dedication.

Are you emotionally ready? You need to take stock of your emotional readiness before getting pregnant again. If you still feel overwhelmed and exhausted by dealing with your first born then this probably isn't the time to get pregnant again. There will come a time when you look around and your house is in order, your child is happy, your relationship with your spouse has returned to a somewhat normal status, and you feel ready to take on a new baby. You may want to approach the subject with your spouse somewhat gingerly since he may be taking a big sigh of relief lately that everything seems to have become less chaotic. There is a chance too that your spouse may be the one to bring it up with you. It's a conversation that needs to take place, though, because you need to be on the same page about your expectations for future pregnancies.

Don't sugar-coat what it's like to have a newborn. There is a saying about what it's like to bring a second baby home: "one is one, and three is three, but two is three." You have gotten into a groove with your baby and when another baby is brought into the equation you will find it hard to juggle in the beginning, especially if your children are close in age. The dreaded "two in diapers" can be a bit of a challenge, although some find it harder to have one in diapers and the other potty-trained. If you're wondering why, then just imagine holding a baby in one arm and trying to balance a toddler on the potty with the other arm. At any rate, you need to recall the sleepless nights and extreme exhaustion that can be associated with a newborn. Don't fool yourself into thinking that all your newborn will do is sleep and allow you and your first-born to go about business as usual. Take into consideration all the factors associated with a pregnancy too. What happens if your doctor puts you on bed rest? Will you have the resources to stay in bed while your first-born putters along alone? Try to take everything into account before getting pregnant again. Of course, for some women, there is simply no perfect time to have a baby and when it happens it's just meant to be. Either way, you'll muddle through no matter what the circumstances . . . moms always do!

Are you all done? Some people make the conscious decision to only have one child. This decision shouldn't be made right after your first baby is born since you're probably in the grips of hormonal surges and exhaustion. If you and your spouse have made an educated decision to not have any more children there are a few options you can explore. You can explore the option of sterilizing yourself, but this is major surgery and brings with it some risk. Your husband might want to look into the option of having a vasectomy. Vasectomies aren't major surgeries, although many men have a lot of apprehension when the subject is brought up because naturally they don't want doctors fiddling around down there. You can also simply stay on birth control or utilize condoms, but birth control can't be used indefinitely and condoms can get boring really quickly. There's always abstinence but most married couples aren't willing to explore this avenue. You should do some research and have a chat with your doctor about which option works best for you.

AGE DIFFERENCES AND SIBLING RIVALRY

Do you want a helper? If you have another baby before your first-born is to a developmental stage where he can help you then you know you'll be in for double work. Even the youngest toddlers can help in one way or another, whether it is grabbing diapers or toys or even dancing and jumping to amuse the new baby. You will be amazed at how amusing your first-born is to your second-born. Even the simple act of your first-born laughing can throw your newborn into hysterical laughter, and this can certainly act as a nice distracter when you need 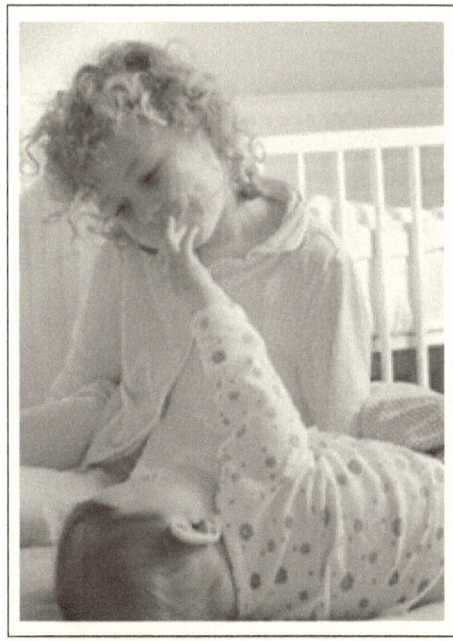 to finish folding laundry. If your first-born is old enough then they can be a massive help to you by grabbing items for you and even helping in diaper changing duties. No matter how old your first-born is, though, it's important to not leave them in complete charge of the newborn, at least not for a while.

A fourteen-year-old first-born may be able to handle babysitting duties but a four-year-old first-born is not ready to handle taking care of a baby solo. Use your best judgment when you decide how much your first-born can help.

Suddenly not being the only show in town can be a shocker. Some researchers suggest the best time to have a baby to avoid major sibling rivalry issues is when your first-born is either younger than eighteen months or older than three years. Younger than eighteen months and they aren't too terribly set in their ways as sibling-free, and older than three is when they are supposed to cognitively be able to understand what is going on when a new baby comes home. Despite what researchers say, though, a lot of the issues regarding sibling rivalry will vary depending upon your first-born's temperament and also with how much you prepare your first-born for the new arrival. There are all sorts of great books and videos, which introduce the concept of new babies joining the family, and of course it is important for you to ready your first-born for the impeding change. Think about it; for all your first-born's life he has been the center of attention and only needed to share toys with occasional playmates. Bring into the equation a screaming newborn that interrupts everyone's sleep and demands a lot of mom and dad's time, and your first-born is bound to be confused and upset. Do your best to make sure that your first-born, no matter what age, is somewhat prepared for the new arrival. After your next baby is born you also need to take care to make sure that your first-born is getting plenty of attention and alone time with you. Although you will probably be exhausted from dealing with your newborn your first child needs you just as much attention from you, if not more so in some cases.

Allow time for adjustment. Depending on the age of your first-born, he will probably display some behaviors, which you hadn't seen before after a new baby joins the family. Younger first-borns may show aggressive tendencies which you have never seen before, and this can either be a product of frustration or out of a genuine curiosity to find out what happens when the newborn gets pinched. A newborn's wail may seem like an interesting reward to an inquisitive toddler. You may also notice some behavior, which is best described as regressive. You first-born may want to use a pacifier or may start speaking in baby talk because they see the attention these actions get the new baby. If your first-born was potty-trained prior to the new baby being born you might find a regression towards wanting to wear diapers again. It is pretty safe to assume that your first-born will eventually work out of these phases, but until then you need to make sure to shower him with plenty of love and attention. As a side note, be sure not to force potty training or any other big changes, such as moving out of a crib and into a big-kid bed, right before the new baby is born or soon thereafter. You will come up against great resistance.

There is certainly something to be said about having babies close together in age because they can grow up playing with the same toys and enjoying the same things. Having children far apart has its merits too since you can concentrate on each child on a more individual level and older children can help a lot too. The choice is ultimately up to you and your partner.

NOW THAT YOU'RE AN EXPERT . . . .

You'll probably realize pretty early on that your baby can melt your heart with a simple giggle. You may be amazed how cleaning up poop and pee becomes commonplace even if the sight of such things made you gag prior to becoming a parent. Yes, having a baby changes your perspective on life in astounding ways. If at times you find yourself feeling a bit inadequate as a parent just take a step back and ask yourself if your baby is receiving unconditional love from you around the clock. If the answer is yes, then you are one fantastic parent. Your baby is just as lucky to have you as you are to have him.

PrivateRights.com

Disclaimer: PrivateRights.com developed these e-books to provide access to valuable information. Although we make every effort to offer only accurate information, we cannot guarantee that the information we make available is always correct or current. PrivateRights.com does not warrant or make any representations as to the quality, content, accuracy, or completeness of the information, text, graphics, links and other items contained in these e-books. Consequently, no one should rely upon any information contained herein, nor make any decisions or take any action based on such information. PrivateRights.com or any subsidiaries are not responsible for any action taken in reliance on the information contained herein and for any damages incurred, whether directly or indirectly, as a result of errors, omissions or discrepancies contained herein.

Full Terms and Conditions can be found at
http://www.PrivateRights.com/TermsandConditions.html

www.ingramcontent.com/pod-product-compliance
Lightning Source LLC
Chambersburg PA
CBHW020351290526
45785CB00005B/2229